Speech, Language, and Hearing Disorders

Speech, Language, and Hearing Disorders

A Guide for the Teacher

Third Edition

Barbara J. Hall
Metropolitan School District of Warren County, Indiana

Herbert J. Oyer
The Ohio State University

William H. Haas
Florida State University

Allyn and Bacon
Boston • London • Toronto • Sydney • Tokyo • Singapore

Executive Editor: Stephen D. Dragin
Series Editorial Assistant: Barbara Strickland
Marketing Manager: Rick Muhr

Copyright © 2001 by Allyn & Bacon
A Pearson Education Company
Needham Heights, MA 02494

Internet: www.abacon.com

Library of Congress Cataloging-in-Publication Data

Hall, Barbara J.
    Speech, language, and hearing disorders : a guide for the teacher / Barbara J. Hall,
  Herbert J. Oyer, William H. Haas (no date).—3rd ed.
      p.   cm.
    Oyer's name appears first as main entry of 2nd ed.
    Includes bibliographical references and index.
    ISBN 0-205-31890-8
      1. Speech disorders in children—United States.   2. Language disorders in
  children—United States. 3. Hearing disorders in children—United States. I. Oyer, Herbert
  J.   II. Haas, William H.   III. Title.
LB3454.H24 2000
371.91'42—dc21   00-038617

Printed in the United States of America

10 9 8 7 6 5 4 3 2 1   04 03 02 01 00

We dedicate the third edition of this book first to the school-age children and youth who have speech, language, and hearing disabilities, and in particular to those whom we have had the privilege of serving. Lessons learned and insights derived therefrom have been of inestimable value.

We also recognize the teachers and parents whose support in the classroom, on the playground, and at home has made possible the success that the students have enjoyed.

Indeed, our dedicatory spirit transcends professional relationships to embrace personal ones as well—to those who encouraged us with patience and understanding. Dr. Hall thanks Bob, Tammy, and Debbie; Dr. Oyer thanks Jane; Dr. Haas thanks Ann.

Contents

Preface

Like the two earlier editions, the third edition of this book holds fast to the original intent of the authors, namely, to provide the information about speech, language, and hearing disorders that is needed by those who are preparing to become teachers and by those who are already teachers. However, this book should also be helpful to anyone who wishes to achieve a better understanding of the communication process and the disorders of communication frequently observed in school-age children. It is our hope that the reader will find the information provided in this book a useful, practical guide to understanding and appreciating the many complexities involved in the communication disorders of children.

The focus of this book was originally determined by the questions asked by approximately 250 teachers and education majors when they responded to our inquiries about what challenges they faced with school-age children who had speech, language, and/or hearing problems. We have continued to ask teachers what they want and need to know. Accordingly, we have provided updated information about the various disorders discussed in the first two editions as well as on topics such as federal laws and regulations that affect speech, language, and hearing programs in the schools. Moreover, because of the federally led initiative toward inclusion and the fact that we are educating more children with disabilities and more children with more severe disabilities in the regular classroom, we have also included basic information about more of the low-incidence populations in which speech, language, and/or hearing are affected, such as children who have tracheostomies and are ventilator-dependent. We have also striven to provide more practical information that teachers can utilize to help children with speech, language, and hearing disabilities to achieve the best communication possible.

At the end of each chapter there is a brief summary along with case histories of children we have known. So that readers may evaluate their understanding of the materials presented, each chapter also has a self-testing section with the answers provided in Appendix B. Of special note is the bibliography of children's books related to speech, language, and hearing in Appendix A. Many of these books are about children who have communication disabilities. Suggestions for using these books are provided in the introduction to the appendix.

The authors wish to acknowledge the work of all of those sources we have cited and from whom we have drawn current clinical concepts and impressions as we developed the third edition of this book. We also wish to express our gratitude to those who have formally or informally made suggestions about the form and substance of the manuscript throughout the revision of this work.

The authors wish to express their gratitude to the following reviewers for their comments on this edition of our book: Norman J. Lass, West Virginia University, and Terre Blankenship, Wichita State University.

About the Authors

Dr. Barbara J. (Crowe) Hall earned both her bachelor's and master's degrees from Purdue University and her doctorate from The Ohio State University. She has worked with both children and adults with a variety of communication disorders in various settings, including schools, hospitals, and university clinics. She has also taught in college—one of her favorite courses is the one for which this book is written. She has presented workshops and papers at state and national meetings. Recently she returned to the public school system, where she works primarily with preschoolers and elementary students. Dr. Hall is especially concerned with the effect communication problems have on how children are perceived by other children and adults. How negative are the perceptions, when do they emerge, and how can they be modified or improved?

Dr. Herbert J. Oyer has worked in a professional capacity as a speech-language pathologist and audiologist in public schools, hospitals, and university clinics. Early in his career he taught in a public school classroom after receiving a bachelor's degree at Bluffton College. Upon completing a master's degree at Bowling Green State University, he taught there and also served in public schools as a speech and hearing clinician. Dr. Oyer completed the Ph.D. degree at The Ohio State University and continued as a faculty member there. He later undertook teaching, clinical, research, and administrative assignments at Michigan State University, where he received the Distinguished Faculty Award. He served as president of the Michigan Speech and Hearing Association and has received Association Honors. He is a past president of the Michigan Academy of Science, Arts, and Letters. As a Fellow of the American Speech, Language, Hearing Association, Dr. Oyer received its highest award, the Honors of the Association. He has served as vice-president of the International Association of Logopedics and Phoniatrics. He has authored/co-authored or edited/co-edited 10 books and over 65 articles in the field. He remains active in research, writing, and consulting.

Dr. William H. Haas received his Ph.D. degree from Michigan State University in 1970. He began his professional career as a public school speech-language pathologist and later directed programs with special emphasis for children with hearing impairment. He is professor emeritus with the College of Communication at Florida State University. Previously he served as a professor of communication disorders, chair of the department of Communication Disorders, and dean of the College of Communication. He holds the Certificate of Clinical Competence in both audiology and speech-language pathology from the American Speech-Language-Hearing Association, is a Fellow with the American Academy of Audiology and the International Collegium of Rehabilitative Audiology, and was awarded Distinguished Alumni status by the College of Communication Arts and Sciences at Michigan State University in 1988. Dr. Haas has presented numerous research papers and workshops on aural rehabilitation.

Speech, Language, and Hearing Disorders

Chapter 1

Introduction to Speech, Language, and Hearing Problems in the Schools

The purpose of this book is to provide you, the teacher or education major, with information that will enable you to understand and promote the speech and language development of all children in your classroom and, in particular, to help children who have speech, language, or hearing disabilities. Each year the number of children with all types of disabilities increases (Karr, 1999; Peters-Johnson, 1998). Over all, slightly more than 10 percent of elementary and secondary students receive special education services. Approximately 50 percent of these children are labeled learning disabled. The next largest category, accounting for approximately another 20 percent, includes children with only speech and language disorders. Slightly more elementary students, age 6 through 11, are labeled with a disability than are secondary students, age 12 through 17 (Peters-Johnson, 1998). Furthermore, not only are we educating more children with disabilities, but we are also educating children with more severe disabilities than ever before. With the federally led initiative for inclusion, all teachers will have children with disabilities in their classrooms, including children with mild to severe communication problems.

Of concern in this book are the approximately 20 percent of children with disabilities who have only speech and language disabilities as well as those children who have some other primary disability, such as mental handicap, visual impairment, hearing impairment, emotional handicap, or other health impairment, and who also exhibit speech and language disabilities. Approximately 50 percent of children who have some other primary disability also have speech-language disabilities. Approximately two thirds of the children whom the speech-language pathologist works with are boys. The speech-language difficulties vary from mild, to moderate, to severe. Approximately 25 percent of communication handicaps are considered to be mild in severity, 50 percent moderate, and 20 percent severe (Peters-Johnson, 1997).

Communication affects every aspect of a person's life: educational achievement, social and psychological development, and vocational success. The specialists who are trained to help these children and to work with other school personnel in their efforts to help them are the speech-language pathologist and the audiologist or educational audiologist.

Who Is the Speech-Language Pathologist?

Over the years this professional has been referred to by many names, including speech teacher, speech correctionist, speech therapist, speech and hearing therapist, speech clinician, speech and language clinician, communication disorders specialist, and speech-language pathologist. The American Speech-Language-Hearing Association (ASHA), the professional organization for those working in the fields of speech-language pathology and audiology, currently recognizes *speech-language pathologist* as the term of choice. However, the terms *speech clinician*, *speech therapist*, and *speech teacher* are still frequently used in the schools.

The goal of the speech-language pathologist is to identify, evaluate, and help people with communicative problems either to correct their problems or to achieve their maximum communicative potential, which may involve compensatory techniques and/or augmentative equipment. In schools the speech-language pathologist is not only involved in working with children with speech and language disabilities but also may serve children with hearing impairments if an educational audiologist is not available.

The speech-language pathologist in the public schools must hold at least a bachelor's degree and teacher certification in speech-language pathology. However, in most states a master's degree is also required. The master's degree as well as national certification and/or state licensure (most states have state licensure or a similar process for regulating the practice of speech-language pathology and audiology) are required for work in all other settings, such as hospitals, private practice, corporations, skilled nursing facilities, universities, community clinics, and rehabilitation centers.

Who Is the Audiologist?

An *audiologist* is the professional who has been trained to understand sound and the science of hearing as well as to diagnose and treat hearing disorders. A certified audiologist has at least a master's degree. Soon many audiologists will hold a new degree called a doctorate of audiology; this degree will be abbreviated AuD. To be certified as an audiologist, the minimum degree by 2007 will be the AuD (New Proposed AuD Standards Published, 1997). The educational audiologist not only works with students with hearing problems but also helps teachers with classroom modifications for children with both temporary and permanent hearing losses.

Do Speech-Language Pathologists and Educational Audiologists Belong to the NEA?

Many who work in the schools do. Many will also belong to ASHA. As the professional organization for audiologists and speech-language pathologists, ASHA advocates not only for these professionals but also for those who have speech, language, or hearing disabilities. ASHA publishes a code of ethics and position statements on almost every aspect of the fields of speech-language pathology and audiology. ASHA is also the national credentialing organization for speech-language pathologists and audiologists. The *Certificate of Clinical Competence* can be earned in audiology (CCC-A) and/or speech-language pathology (CCC-SLP) through earning bachelor's and master's degrees from accredited programs of study, passing a national examination, and successfully completing a year of supervised work following the master's degree. During the master's program, students will complete two externships, one in the schools (which is very similar to student teaching for education majors) and one in a health-based setting. Slightly over half of the certified speech-language pathologists who work full-time work in the public schools (*School Services: Answers to Frequently Asked Questions*, 1998).

Besides advocacy and credentialing, ASHA is also involved in:

- Publishing several refereed journals. Refereed journals are journals whose articles have been peer-reviewed for standards of quality.
- Providing many avenues for continuing education, including conferences, videoconferences, and teleseminars.
- Recruitment and retention. According to statistics published by the U.S. Department of Labor, job opportunities for speech-language pathologists will increase by more than 50 percent through 2006 (Job Opportunities Ahead for Speech-Language Pathologists, Audiologists, 1998). ASHA is also concerned about the low percentage of its members who are bilingual.
- Sponsoring special interest sections, such as Language, Learning, and Education; Hearing and Hearing Disorders in Childhood; and Communication Disorders and Sciences in Culturally and Linguistically Diverse Populations. Some of these groups work with other professional organizations, such as the American Psychological Association, on issues like position statements and advocacy.
- Sponsoring specialty recognition programs that help to identify those professionals who have specialized in a narrowly defined area, such as fluency, rather than in the overall field of communication.
- Sponsoring the National Student Speech-Hearing-Language Association (NSSHLA) and the National Black Association for Speech-Language and Hearing (NBASLH).

- Sponsoring research. ASHA is particularly concerned about research on the efficacy, effectiveness, outcomes, and costs of services (Amiot, 1998; Baum, 1998; Gallagher, Swigert, & Baum, 1998; Logemann, 1998; Seymour, 1997). This type of research can be applied to all classroom teaching methods.
- Keeping members up to date on laws and the regulations based on those laws.

Are There Speech-Language Pathology Aides (Like Teacher Aides)?

Yes, in many states. However, they are not permitted in all states. The terms *aides, paraprofessionals, service extenders, speech-language pathology assistants,* and *supportive personnel* are used interchangeably. The aide must work under the supervision of a speech-language pathologist or audiologist. Some states, such as Ohio, license these individuals, while in other states they are hired under the classification of teacher aides. Some institutions of higher learning offer associate degrees for those wanting to become a speech-language assistant.

Speech-language pathologists and audiologists are seeing larger numbers of children and youth and many of these have more complicated problems. Just as in the classroom, aides enable speech-language pathologists to do more without sacrificing quality of instruction. Also, aides who are bilingual and can help work with children who speak English as a second language (ESL) are invaluable in communicating with the children, parents, and the community of foreign speakers at-large. The same is true of bidialectical paraprofessionals.

The state of Ohio specifies that "an aide shall work under the direction and supervision of a speech-language pathologist or audiologist licensed by the board," and that "they shall not work independently" (*Ohio Law and Rules Governing Speech-Language Pathology and Audiology Aides*). The initial cost for aide licensure is $100, with a biennial renewal fee of $50. In order to obtain licensure, the individual must be a high school graduate and file an approved plan of work in conjunction with and signed by the speech-language pathologist or audiologist who is going to supervise the work, noting the location of anticipated employment, a description of the duties, and the nature of the direct supervision to be received. Furthermore, there are numerous proscriptions; for example, an aide may not perform diagnostic testing. An identifying badge must also be worn in the workplace. ASHA has been encouraged to develop credentialing standards for aides because of concerns about the viability of both the concept and the procedures associated with the licensing of aides by states.

Does Every School Have a Speech-Language Pathologist?

One of the first public school "speech correction" (as it was then called) programs began in Chicago in 1910, with several of the larger, urban school districts following in the next decade (Moore & Kester, 1953). The number of children served, especially in small and rural districts, expanded tremendously during the 1950s and 1960s. Today, in order to comply with federal and state laws, the answer is a resounding "yes." Most school districts hire their own speech-language pathologists, but some districts contract with a private practice, which may be a fairly large entity or one speech-language pathologist set up in an individual practice.

Sometimes finding speech-language pathologists is difficult because of a shortage, especially in rural areas that have a low population density and rugged or dangerous terrain. To complicate matters, these areas are often populated by people representing a cultural and/or linguistic diversity. Legally, however, a shortage of speech-language pathologists is not an excuse for not providing services. Therefore, some unique solutions have been tried, such as multiple agencies working together and long-distance hearing screening (Coleman, Thompson-Smith, Pruitt, & Richards, 1999).

What Does Federal Law Have to Do with Speech-Language Pathology and Audiology?

The first federal laws concerning the education of children with disabilities were passed in the 1960s, first dealing with educating children in state-supported institutions and then at the local education agency level. However, it was PL 94-142, entitled the Education for All Handicapped Children Act of 1975 (EHA), that heralded a big change and many ensuing laws involving not only school-age children and youth but also the 0–5 population.

PL refers to Public Law. The number preceding the hyphen represents the session of Congress during which the law was passed, and the number following the hyphen represents the number of the law passed in that session. Therefore, PL 94-142 was the 142nd law passed by the 94th session of Congress. All laws are printed in volumes entitled the *United States Statutes at Large*, and the regulations relating to the laws can be found in the *Federal Register*.

PL 94-142 mandated that all children with disabilities receive a free education appropriate to their needs. Although some children with disabilities were receiving an education before the enactment of this law, over one million were not. Of those being serviced, it was estimated that over one-half were not receiving an appropriate education. Before Congress acted, state and local educational agencies had the option of providing or not providing education to the disabled. PL 94-142 addressed the needs of children with disabilities, regardless of the degree of severity, between the ages of 3 and 21. Exceptions to age inclusions were granted in states where state laws, regulations, or court orders were in conflict with PL 94-142, and then children below age 5 and above age 18 were excluded. Each state had to enact its own legislation, rules, and regulations to comply with PL 94-142.

PL 99-457, the Education of the Handicapped Act Amendments of 1986, no longer gave the states a choice about providing services to children from age 3 to kindergarten enrollment. It also provided incentives to states to serve newborns to 3-year-olds.

In 1990, with the passage of PL 101-476, the title of the Education of the Handicapped Act, which included PL 94-142 and PL 99-457, was changed to *Individuals with Disabilities Education Act (IDEA)*. This law was updated in 1997 with PL 105-17, the Individuals with Disabilities Education Act Amendments, which funded special education for five million children with various disabilities. The last regulations of this act became effective during 1999.

It was felt that children with disabilities were not being challenged to succeed and reach their potential functioning and that an unnecessary and inequitable gap existed between what children with disabilities were expected to learn and what their "normal" peers were expected to learn. Therefore, the thrust of current legislation is to allow all students to participate and succeed in the general education curriculum in the regular education environment to the maximum extent possible. Historically, the term *least restrictive environment* has been used to refer to the most "normal" or "regular" setting in which a child can function for the school day or for a portion of the school day, and the term *mainstreaming* has been commonly used to describe this process in which children are with their normal peers for as much of the day as possible. The more current term is *inclusion*, meaning that children with disabilities are included in the regular curriculum and the regular classroom. There are monies available through IDEA for making sure that all concerned are knowledgeable about the law and for research to identify how best to teach the regular educational curriculum to children with disabilities in the regular classroom. Whenever a child is not participating in regular education in the classroom, an explanation of why and to what extent must be included in the individualized educational program (IEP). Some important issues and highlights of the legislation that affects children with disabilities are as follows.

An *IEP* must be completed for each child with a disability. "Education" refers not just to academic achievement, but to social, emotional, and vocational achievement as well. The focus is to be on the general education curriculum, which is thought to prepare the child more completely for employment and independent living.

The IEP team, the people who design and write the IEP, must include the parents, at least one regular education teacher if the child participates at all in the regular educational environment, and at least one special education provider. An administrator, others who have worked with the child, professionals outside of the school system who provide services to the child, and sometimes the child complete the team. IEP meetings must take place at least every 12 months, more often if needed or requested. Meetings must be arranged at mutually convenient times for both the school and parents. Notification of the meeting must be sent to all participants early enough so that schedules can be arranged in order for everyone to attend. This includes the school arranging for substitutes so that teachers can attend meetings during the school day. If more than one regular education teacher works with a child, then one such teacher may be designated as the IEP team participant, and that teacher should obtain input from the other regular education teachers. When there is an insurmountable scheduling problem, the law does allow for telephone or video conferences. Sometimes IEP meetings are held during summer months so that service can be in place when the school year begins.

Based on evaluations and descriptions of the child's current level of functioning within the educational setting, the child is given a "label" or category designation, such as mental handicap, vision impairment, orthopedic handicap, hearing impairment, or communication handicap. The decision regarding educational placement may not be made on the basis of the disability. Decisions to provide services and which services must always be made on a case-by-case basis, not because the child belongs to a particular disability category.

With input from all members, including the parents, the team considers the impact of the student's disability on the child's ability to progress in the general education curriculum and identifies the child's strengths and areas of need. These strengths and needs are identified from evaluation results and from information gleaned from working with or teaching the child. Using the identified needs as a basis, annual goals are written that will allow the child to participate and progress in the general education curriculum as well as in social, emotional, and vocational areas. Short-term objectives or benchmarks that will facilitate the child's achieving the annual goals are then written. The projected date for initiation of services and the frequency and duration of services are decided. Also included are the person(s) responsible for each objective, dates for anticipated initiation of work toward each objective, and how success on each objective will be measured. There are not endless pages of tedious goals and objectives, but broader areas that focus on modifications, accommodations, equipment, related services, and support for school personnel that are necessary for the child to be successful in the general education curriculum. Unless the IEP team documents needs that preclude inclusion, the child will be educated with children who have no disabilities and within the classroom that he or she would attend if not disabled.

The term *assistive technology* is often used and is defined as any product or piece of equipment, such as a hearing aid, communication board, or hand-held calculator, that increases a child's functional capabilities. Assistive technology services are any services that help a child select, acquire, or use an assistive technology device. It should be noted that school-purchased equipment must be allowed to go home with the child if the IEP team deems that the child needs access to the device in order to receive a *free and appropriate education (FAPE)*.

Progress on the goals and short-term objectives is reported to the parents at least as often as regular report cards go out. One easy way to report progress is to use the IEP form and note, for example, whether the goal has been achieved, progress made but goal not achieved, no progress made, or goal achieved but not maintained.

The IEP team also decides if the child will participate in state-wide or district-wide assessments and, if so, whether there will be any accommodations, such as longer testing time or having portions of the test read to the child, or if the child will instead participate in some other sort of assessment. Functional assessments, designed to be more outcome-focused, may be used as alternatives. These assessments may look at areas such as the extent to which progress in academic areas depends on supports not provided to other students, the degree to which the student engages in social relationships, the degree of independence in the restroom and the cafeteria, the degree to which the child follows school rules without reminders from adults, and the amount of support necessary for completing academic work.

Another decision made by the IEP team is whether or not to recommend an extended school year. This decision is based on factors such as the chances of the child's regression, past history of regression, the child's degree of disability, and the parents' ability to work with the child and/or reinforce past instruction at home.

When there are disagreements about the child's disability, placement, educational goal and objectives, or any other aspect of the IEP, mediation services must be offered at no charge to the parents. Parents have further legal rights that must be explained to them by the school district.

Children cannot be denied services based solely on disciplinary issues, if the problem is related to the child's disability. Children with behavior problems should have behavior plans that are a part of their IEPs.

All teachers who work with the child, and anyone else, such as an aide or school nurse, who is responsible for any part of the IEP implementation must have access to a copy of the IEP. All are responsible for understanding their responsibilities and the modifications, accommodations, and other supports that are provided for in the IEP.

Before the IDEA Amendments were passed, triennial (every 3 years) reevaluations were required. There is now some flexibility, and, based upon IEP team members' input, a review of the existing data rather than a reevaluation may be sufficient for deciding that the disability still exists and that services are still needed and should be continued. The regular education teacher, as well as special education staff, will need to be prepared with evidence to support their positions.

Transitional services must be provided for vocational training, postsecondary education, continuing education, or independent community living if the student is over age 16.

Special notice should be taken of children and families who do not speak English or for whom English is a second language. All evaluations must be performed in the child's native language as well as in English. All correspondence, written and oral, with the parents must be in the parents' customary language.

Children who do not qualify for services under IDEA may receive help under *Section 504* of the Rehabilitation Act of 1973. Children covered by Section 504 may have a mental or physical disability that substantially limits a major life activity, such as walking, hearing, speaking, seeing, breathing, learning, working, or self-care. Many children with attention deficit disorder (ADD) can qualify to receive help under Section 504. Other laws that might be of interest and which the reader might want to investigate further include the Americans with Disabilities Act (ADA) passed in 1990, Goals 2000: Educate America Act of 1993, and Improving America's Schools Act (IASA) passed in 1994.

Back to communication: How does federal law relate to speech-language pathology and audiology? Every school-age child who is identified as having a communication disorder that adversely affects educational achievement falls under the jurisdiction of the law. An IEP must be completed and appropriate services given. If the child qualifies for another special education program, speech and language services are regarded as related services. The speech-language pathologist may be a part of the IEP team. However, if the child qualifies only for speech or language services, the speech-language pathologist is the only special education staff on the IEP team, and these services are considered special education and, as such, are eligible for federal funding. Understanding the funding issue allows school personnel to help parents understand why their child is categorized as a special education student, especially if their child's problem is relatively minor, such as a "w" for "r" substitution.

If a child has only a communication disorder involving a problem like voice quality, speech sound substitutions, stuttering, or language, the regular education teacher still has obligations at the IEP meeting. For example, the regular education teacher will be called upon to explain how speech sound errors (e.g., "w" for "r" as in "wabbit" for "rabbit") affect oral reading or speaking activities within the classroom or on the playground. Does it make the child hard to understand? Do other children tease? In providing input to the IEP, the speech-language pathologist will work to integrate goals and objectives with the general education curriculum.

Speech-language pathologists working in the schools also evaluate and provide services to preschoolers. Instead of, but very similar to, an IEP, an individualized family service plan (IFSP) is completed for children up to age 3. The major difference is the focus on the family; the goals to be achieved are for both the child and the family, and services are offered to both.

Are There Differences in the Terms Communication, Language, and Speech?

Communication. Language. Speech. These three terms are interchangeable for many people. However, for the purposes of this book, distinctions will need to be made among them.

Communication, the most general of the terms, implies a transfer of knowledge, ideas, opinions, and feelings. Most often this transfer is via language. However, there are other means. For example, body language can be a powerful tool of communication, although most linguists would not be willing to classify body language as an example of a formal language because it is nonlinguistic in nature, involving body movements like pointing, waving, fidgeting, and facial expressions rather than the signs and symbols of a language. Communication between an infant and its caregiver is present at birth even though the infant has not yet learned to use language or speech (Matthews, 1986).

Language, a more specific term, can be defined simply as a formalized method of communication consisting of (1) the signs and symbols by which ideas can be represented, and (2) the rules governing these signs and symbols (e.g., how the symbols can be combined). Language occurs among a community of language users, which means that the person or persons receiving it must have shared meanings attached to the message content. Language is unique to humans because only human beings are able to use language to communicate about the past and the future as well as the present (Bolton, 1981). There are several modes by which humans may communicate their language, including reading, writing, speaking, and listening. These modes can be classified either as receptive or expressive language. Reading and listening are examples of receptive language (i.e., the message is received and decoded or interpreted). Writing and speaking are forms of expressive language whereby the message is encoded or produced.

Speech, the narrowest of the terms, is the vocal or spoken production of language and, as such, is the fastest and most efficient means of communicating. It can be defined as the motor production of speech sounds (i.e., the individual consonant and vowel sounds). Speech sounds have rules governing their use and combination. Motor production involves the movements made by the various parts of the body in order to produce sound waves that travel through the air, eventually impinging upon the listener's ears. Motor production of speech sounds will be referred to as *articulation*.

What Kinds of Communicative Disorders Should the Teacher Look for in the Classroom?

This question might be divided into two questions, one dealing with speech and one with language (hearing impairments are dealt with in Chapter 7). One could first ask what kinds of speech problems are there, or how can the teacher determine when a child might have a speech problem and when should a child be referred to the speech-language pathologist?

For years the standard definition in the field of speech-language pathology has been that speech is abnormal when it is conspicuous, unintelligible, or unpleasant; interferes with communication; or causes the speaker to be maladjusted (Van Riper & Emerick, 1984). In other words, the listener is so intrigued with *how* the message is being communicated that attention is drawn away from *what* is being communicated. However, the definition makes it clear that individual circumstances, such as the speaker's age, cultural norms, and environment, also must be considered. For example, a 3-year-old child is not expected to articulate (produce speech sounds) as well as a 10-year-old child or an adult. We would not tend to be distracted from the content of the message "I'm goin' to dreth up like a thkeleton for Halloween" if we were talking to a 3-year-old, but we might be if we were talking to a 10-year-old. In some localities, words such as "runnin'" for "running," "warsh" for "wash," and even "dese" and "dem" for "these" and "them" are quite acceptable and are unnoticed in that environment, but they would certainly be noticed on the six o'clock news.

Problems that are labeled as abnormal speech are typically placed in one or more of the following categories:

- Speech Sound Disorders: These problems involve both articulatory disorders and phonological disorders. *Articulation* refers to the motor ability to produce speech sounds, while *phonology* involves acquisition of the abstract linguistic rules that govern speech sounds. More detail will be presented in chapters 2 and 7.

- Fluency Disorders: Fluency problems are characterized by repetitions, prolongations, or blocks that interrupt the flow or rhythm of speech to an abnormal degree and are further discussed in Chapter 4.
- Voice Disorders: Deviations in pitch, pitch patterns, range of pitch, vocal quality (words such as "hoarse," "nasal," and "breathy" help describe disorders of vocal quality), loudness, or loudness patterns constitute voice disorders. Sometimes such deviations are not pleasant to listen to and often are not appropriate for the age or sex of the speaker. These are covered in chapters 5 and 7.

What kinds of language impairments are there? Briefly, they involve problems in one or more of the dimensions or components of language: (1) syntax, (2) semantics, (3) morphology, (4) pragmatics, and (5) phonology. The first four are discussed in Chapter 3; phonology is examined in Chapter 2.

What Causes Speech and Language Problems?

Causes vary and are not always known. Attempts are made to determine the cause(s) of any particular disorder so that if the source of the problem is still present, it can be eliminated or corrected. If the cause cannot be rectified, it may be possible to improve communication by teaching compensatory techniques. On the other hand, if the cause cannot be determined, it is very likely that speech therapy can still be successful. Speech and language are complicated processes. To communicate vocally, the speaker must possess certain physical prerequisites, including neurological integrity. Causes will be dealt with for each specific disorder in the following chapters. However, in general it should be noted that factors associated with communication disorders as well as other disorders include variables such as lack of adequate prenatal care, substance abuse, teenage pregnancy, premature birth, poverty, lack of family and social support systems, parents who are members of socially dysfunctional families, abuse, craniofacial anomalies, child's medical needs not being met, child's lack of stimulation, genetics, and hearing loss. Two of these factors (genetics and hearing loss) deserve a very basic introduction here, although they will also be discussed in other chapters in more detail.

More and more research is indicating that genetics may play a part in communication disorders. Some are manifested at birth, such as Down syndrome and cleft palate. Some geneticists feel that direct genetic manipulation may be feasible in the twenty-first century. British researchers have identified a gene area that affects human speech (Porterfield, 1998), and others feel that there may be a genetic link in some cases to phonology disorders (Research Conference Highlights Advances in Genetics Research, 1996; Uffen, 1997). Genetics also play a role in stuttering and some types of hearing impairments.

Through hearing, children learn to decode the language spoken in their environment. Unless they learn the basics of their language by age 6 or 7, they may never become proficient in any language. Thus, it is imperative that infants with hearing loss be identified. Currently the average age at which hearing loss is diagnosed is 2½ years, well into the critical period for learning speech and language (New Bill Supports Early Identification of Hearing Loss, 1999). This is particularly sad because hearing loss can be diagnosed within a few hours of birth. To that end, state legislatures and Congress have been introducing and passing newborn hearing screening laws to identify newborns with hearing losses so that intervention may begin immediately (Davolt, 1999a; New Bill Supports Early Identification of Hearing Loss, 1999). The majority of children who are born with hearing impairments are educated in regular school settings (Ross, 1994).

Another cause of hearing loss and possible speech and language delays is *otitis media*, the number one reason for preschoolers to go to a doctor as well as the most common reason for antibiotics being prescribed to children. It has been estimated that 80 percent of all children have had otitis media by their third birthday (Janota, 1999). *Otitis media* is an inflammation of the middle ear. If there is also fluid in the middle ear that is not infected, it is called *otitis media with effusion (OME)*. When infection is present, the term *acute otitis media (AOM)* is used. Symptoms such as irritability, tugging on the ear, complaints of pain, and fever may or may not be present. Often there is a fluctuation between acute otitis media and otitis media with effusion. Fluid in the middle ear may persist for several weeks or months. If the fluid is present for 3 months or longer, the term *chronic otitis media with effusion* is used. The common cold, respiratory viruses, and allergies can play a role in otitis media. Sometimes otitis media with effusion is accompanied by a temporary mild to moderate hearing loss that may fluctuate, with the degree of loss correlating with the quantity of fluid present in the middle ear (Roberts & Medley, 1995). Repeated episodes may cause permanent hearing loss (Who Has Hearing, Speech, and Language Problems?, 1995). Otitis media is two to four times more prevalent in African American children than in Caucasian children (Janota, 1999). Researchers are working on an experimental vaccine to protect against otitis media, but in the meantime there will be children with some form of otitis media in the classroom and some will present with a hearing loss.

Speech, language, and learning may all be affected by the hearing problems associated with otitis media. In school the teacher may not notice any symptoms or the child may appear inattentive or distractible and may seem to have difficulty following directions (which were not fully heard). The child may also seem to have more problems in larger groups and in background noise, but still do well one on one and in quiet settings. Seldom will the child complain about being unable to hear.

In previous years it has been assumed that a unilateral hearing loss (in only one ear versus bilateral, which is in both ears) was probably not educationally significant (English & Church, 1999). However, this view has changed. A unilateral loss may particularly cause difficulty in background noise, and schools are noisy places, as will be further discussed in Chapter 9.

Hearing loss may also be caused by injury; other illnesses, such as German measles (rubella); and loud noises. Montgomery and Fujikawa (1992) provided a review of the literature that indicates there is an increase in high-frequency hearing loss in school-age children due to loud noises, including music, in-the-ear headsets, guns, shop class machinery, and band.

What Are the Responsibilities of the Speech-Language Pathologist?

In this introductory chapter, general responsibilities will be discussed. More specific details will be provided in the other chapters.

Identification and Assessment

Identification involves identifying students who are in need of assessment. Assessment involves the appraisal of the communicative status of an individual in terms of speech and/or language abilities. There are two aspects to assessment: initial assessment, which involves identification and diagnosis; and ongoing assessment, which continues during therapy in order to monitor or evaluate a child's progress. Ongoing assessment during therapy may result in a continuation or a modification of therapeutic techniques or programs. The discussion here will focus on the initial assessment, which is a two-stage process involving screening and an individual assessment or evaluation that results in a diagnosis.

Speech and Language Screening
Screening is a rapid assessment done in order to identify those children who need a complete evaluation. Who is screened will vary from school district to school district and, within some districts, from school building to school building. In some school districts, kindergartners, children new to the school district, teacher referrals, and parent referrals are screened. In other school districts, children may not be screened until they enter the second, third, or even fourth grade, on the assumption that maturity for speech is not complete until age 7, 8, or 9. In yet other districts, no general screening takes place and speech-language pathologists rely solely on referrals from teachers, parents, and other school personnel. Self-referrals, particularly at the secondary level, may also be encouraged.

The practice of relying solely on referrals allows for those in the individual's environment to decide whether a communicative disorder is present (McDermott, 1985). It has been argued that accountability in terms of time and money expended can best be achieved when speech-language pathologists do not screen all students, as most will not exhibit communicative problems (Gantwerk, 1985). This procedure may work very well in school systems in which teachers, other school personnel, and even parents have received training in recognizing and referring children with suspected problems. Phillips (1976) reported on a relationship between the grade taught and awareness of speech disorders in children, with teacher awareness greatest in the lower grades and decreasing as grade taught increased. Yet referrals are often relied on as a means of identification at the secondary level, even when the speech-language pathologist does the screening at the elementary level (Neal, 1976). Therefore, the secondary teacher should strive to be especially cognizant of students with possible speech and language problems.

Screening of nonreferrals takes place throughout the school year, although many speech-language pathologists try to complete as much as possible at the beginning of the school year. The speech-language pathologist assigned to a school building may do all of the screening, or a team of speech-language pathologists in the district may work together to screen an entire school within a day, helping to minimize disruptions. When a child is identified as having no problem, this information is recorded and, depending on screening procedures, the child might not be automatically screened again. This is a time-efficient procedure; however, it has two problems. First, the screenings are rapid, and subtle problems may be missed. Second, some problems, especially fluency and voice problems, may develop later. Therefore, teachers should never be reluctant to refer a child for testing, even when they know that the child previously passed a screening.

According to ASHA, the average screening takes approximately 5 minutes per child (Task Force Report on School Speech, Hearing, and Language Screening Procedures, 1973). Screening of a child immediately identified as needing an individual evaluation may not require 5 minutes, while screening of a child who has no problem may require more than 5 minutes to be sure that a problem is not missed.

The speech-language pathologist may set up the screening in a variety of ways. Frequently a small group of children is taken into a quiet hallway or to a therapy room. Each child may be given a formal screening test and/or be asked to give his or her name, read, describe a picture, name pictures of objects, count, repeat sentences, and answer open-ended questions to elicit a speech and language sample from which the speech-language pathologist will judge intelligibility, articulation, voice, fluency, and language. As the speech-language pathologist finishes with each child, that child may be sent back to the classroom so that another child may leave the room and join the group, or all of the children may return together while a new group joins the speech-language pathologist. This latter procedure saves time because each child (except the first in a group) has an opportunity to observe several other children being tested. The speech-language pathologist may not need to give as many directions and the children may be more relaxed and comfortable in the screening situation. (Task Force Report on School Speech, Hearing, and Language Screening Procedures, 1973). Screening is also sometimes conducted in a corner of the classroom.

Parental permission is not required for screening. However, many school systems, out of courtesy and an interest in good school–parent relationships and in order to comply with state or local policy, will notify parents of upcoming screenings. This notification may provide an impetus to parents who have questioned their child's communicative abilities to contact the speech-language pathologist.

Any child who has been identified as having difficulty in the classroom and has been prereferred to an educational problem-solving team with a name, such as

Child Study Team or Intervention Assistance Team, or who has been referred for a psychoeducational evaluation must also be screened by the speech-language pathologist for speech and language difficulties. These children are also given a hearing screening. It should be noted that referrals must be assessed within the time stipulated by law.

Individual Assessment and Evaluation of Speech and Language

Written parental permission is required by law for an individual assessment. The assessment procedures must be age-appropriate and free of cultural and linguistic bias. The assessment may take up to 2 hours or more and should result in a diagnosis of the child's speech and language status, a statement regarding severity of the problem, a statement regarding impact of the problem on educational performance, and recommendations that can be shared with the IEP committee. It should provide information pertaining to the child's strengths as well as needs and, thus, the goals and objectives that should be considered for a child as well as the kinds of therapeutic techniques that are most apt to be successful with the child. A variety of procedures is involved and, depending on individual circumstances, may include:

1. An oral peripheral examination (a visual determination of whether the oral structures appear to be capable of producing normal speech)
2. An articulation test (an evaluation of the child's ability to produce speech sounds in isolation, words, sentences, and spontaneous speech)
3. A measure of auditory discrimination ability (can the child hear the difference between a correct speech sound and the sound that he or she substitutes for the correct one)
4. A measure of stimulability (can the child produce the sound he or she is asked to produce with or without specific directions; if so, the child is stimulable)
5. Tests of expressive and receptive language skills (using standardized tests as well as an analysis of spontaneous speech)
6. An evaluation of fluency
7. An evaluation of voice
8. A hearing test (although this may legally be the responsibility of the audiologist or school nurse)
9. A case history (obtained from the parents of younger children and possibly from both the child and the parents in the case of older children)
10. An examination of classroom or curriculum-based samples of the child's work
11. Checklists or scales completed by parents and/or those who work with the child in the educational setting

The speech-language pathologist may also want to observe the child in the classroom or on the playground. Additional information, such as the child's cognitive functioning or home environment, that is obtained by other school personnel may be helpful in interpreting the findings.

Hearing Screenings

Hearing screenings may be conducted by the speech-language pathologist, the educational audiologist, or the school nurse. Most states require that the children in certain grades, most typically kindergarten, first, fourth, seventh, and tenth; new children to the district; children with past histories of ear problems; and referrals be screened for hearing loss. A quiet environment is required. When a screening is failed, an audiometric test to determine thresholds is given. These procedures are described in Chapter 7.

Therapy

Therapy is sometimes called *remediation* or *delivery of services*. Therapy may be direct, with the speech-language pathologist working directly with the child, or indirect, with the speech-language pathologist working with others in the child's environment, such as the academic teacher, an aide, or a parent, to enable them to help the child with communication skills.

Service delivery options is a term used to refer to the different methods of providing services. There are a multitude of terms used to describe these methods and little consensus on what most of these terms mean (Blosser & Kratcoski, 1997). ASHA recognizes the following seven service delivery options (Ad Hoc Committee on the Roles and Responsibilities of the School-Based Speech-Language Pathologist, 1999). Readers will find these methods or variations of them in their schools even though they may be referred to by another name.

1. Monitoring: The speech-language pathologist monitors or checks on a student's speech and language performance. This option is frequently used just before a student is dismissed from therapy.

2. Pullout: This is the traditional model in which a student or small group of students is pulled out of the classroom and goes into the speech-language room. This method has also been called *itinerant* and *intermittent direct service*. Those of you reading this book who were once enrolled in speech therapy were probably served via this program. You most likely left the classroom to go to therapy twice a week for 20-to-30-minute sessions. This pullout model includes sessions up to 1 hour long and as often as 5 days a week, depending on the needs of the child. The child may be seen individually or in a small group. ASHA (Guidelines for Caseload Size for Speech-Language Services in the Schools, 1984) recommends that the small group include no more than three children. The teacher and speech-language pathologist may consult with each other so that the speech-language pathologist can incorporate classroom materials into the child's communicative program.

3. Collaborative Consultation: Collaboration involves sharing the same "turf," which individuals on all sides may find difficult. However, it is sometimes necessary for successful educational programming. The speech-language pathologist does not work directly with the child but consults with and helps the teacher(s) and/or parent(s) work with the child to enhance communicative ability.

This method, sometimes called *indirect service*, can be appropriate for children with very mild to rather severe problems. For example, a child who has a stuttering problem may be served via the pullout method until he or she demonstrates the ability to use appropriate "controls" to facilitate fluent speech. The IEP team may choose not to dismiss the child entirely but to continue services via collaborative consultation to ensure that the child has the necessary environmental support to maintain the improved communicative status. At the other end of the severity continuum is a child who physically cannot talk but uses an alternative communication device that involves the use of a computer. The speech-language pathologist plans therapy or intervention, instructs others in carrying it out, and periodically reevaluates progress, modifying the program as necessary. If children can be appropriately served by the consultation model, they should be, because it meets the legal mandate of least restrictive environment.

4. Classroom-Based: This service option is also referred to as *integrated service, curriculum-based, transdisciplinary, interdisciplinary,* and *inclusive programming*. It, too, involves turf sharing. The speech-language pathologist works directly with the child in the classroom or other natural environment, for example, the playground (Guidelines for Caseload Size and Speech-Language Service Delivery in the Schools, 1993). Elksnin and Capilouto (1994) described seven classroom-based delivery approaches: one teaching while one observes, one teaching while one drifts, station teaching, parallel teaching, remedial teaching, supplemental teaching, and team teaching. Even without defining these or describing these in any detail, the reader can get the general idea of how this method could work. Farber and Klein (1999) provide a good description of 10 years of research in this area, along with the pros and cons.

With the classroom-based method it is much easier to integrate communication skills with academic content, such as vocabulary and concepts in the various curriculum areas. This model provides a more natural environment, and so *carryover* (the habitual use in the child's natural environment of what has been taught and learned) may be more quickly and easily achieved. Advocates of this kind of program also presume that the student is less stigmatized by it than by the pullout program.

5. Self-Contained Program: Also called *academically integrated direct service,* this alternative is most frequently used with children who have severe or multiple communicative problems. Such children are placed in a special class for the majority of the school day. They may be mainstreamed for some educational or social (e.g., recess) activities. Unless the class is team taught with a certified academic teacher, the speech-language pathologist must also be certified as a regular education teacher and is responsible for academics as well as speech-language therapy.

6. Community-Based: In this model, therapy is provided outside of the school in the community, most often in the home. This is most frequently used for preschoolers but may be used for school-age children, especially for those who are medically fragile and/or have severe disabilities. Usually there is an extra emphasis on functional skills in a natural environment.

7. Combination: More than one of the above options is utilized. For example, a child may be seen in the classroom two times a week and in a pullout session once a week.

The choice of service delivery method should be based on the needs of the child. Therefore, it would be expected that any one speech-language pathologist would be using more than one service delivery option. It would also be reasonable to expect that more than one kind of service delivery would be used with any one child during that child's tenure in therapy. For example, a pullout program might be followed by a combination pullout/classroom-based, followed by a classroom-based, and ending with a monitoring program. A survey of speech-language pathologists conducted by ASHA (Peters-Johnson, 1996) revealed that the pullout model is used by the majority of school-based speech-language pathologists; the majority of the children are seen in a group rather than individually; and the classroom-based model was used more with children who had needs in the areas of language, augmentative/alternative communication, auditory processing, aural rehabilitation (*aural* refers to hearing), and central auditory processing (to be discussed in Chapter 8).

Why Are Some Children Selected for Therapy and Others Are Not?

School districts should have a set of criteria that must be met before a child is considered communication handicapped and eligible for services. However, this does not mean that a child who is enrolled in speech therapy in School District A would necessarily be enrolled in speech therapy in School District B or C. Each school district can set its own criteria for determining a handicapping condition, although there may be state guidelines that school districts are encouraged to follow. Within the school district's criteria the actual decision concerning disability and provision of services for a particular child rests with the IEP committee. It is important to remember that whether or not a child meets certain arbitrary criteria for language remediation, articulation therapy, et cetera, it is still the prerogative and responsibility of the IEP committee to decide whether or not the child has a disability and does or does not need services.

Will a Child Have Speech-Language Homework?

Some speech-language pathologists regularly assign homework. Others do so on an as-needed basis, and still others never give homework. Some use a weekly folder that goes home with papers either (1) to stay at home, to show the parent what the child is doing and how he or she is progressing and/or to provide materials for the parent to work on with the child at home or (2) to be returned to school, either completed if the papers were homework or signed by the parent to indicate that the parent is aware of what the child is doing. Whether or not there is homework will depend on the specific goals for a particular child.

How Are the Type of Program, Frequency, and Duration of Therapy Determined?

The delivery of services model and the frequency and duration of each therapy session are selected and approved by the IEP committee and are recorded on the child's IEP. It should be emphasized that the model of remediation chosen as the mode for delivery of services should be the model best suited to the needs of the child, not just the most convenient. For example, age and the severity of the disorder should be considered when making decisions about frequency and duration of therapy. Attention span may dictate that two 15-minute sessions per day would be preferable to one 30-minute session (Work, 1985). Many school districts and states not only have guidelines that the IEP committee can consult regarding eligibility for services but also for service delivery options and total numbers of minutes of service based on the type of disability, severity of the disability, and/or age of the child.

What Does the Speech-Language Pathologist Do with the Child, or What Really Goes on in Therapy?

In the succeeding chapters, which focus on particular communicative problems, therapeutic procedures will be briefly described so that the reader has an understanding of the general procedures that may be used for each disorder. Teachers are encouraged to discuss with a speech-language pathologist the possibility of observing a therapy session, particularly a session involving students in their own classrooms. Most speech-language pathologists would eagerly welcome such a request.

When Is a Child Dismissed from Therapy?

Obviously, if the speech-language pathologist felt that a child was performing a new speech or language behavior 100 percent of the time, the child could be dismissed. However, dismissal from therapy is frequently arranged at some point before the 100 percent criterion is reached (generally in the 80–90 percent range), as past experience has shown that children usually continue to make progress after the termination of therapy. Children are also dismissed from therapy when objective measures indicate that they have reached their maximum potential considering their organic, physiological, and/or cognitive status. The IEP or IFSP committee is responsible for making such decisions.

Philosophy of Speech-Language Therapy

A brief comment regarding philosophy of speech-language therapy would be pertinent at this point. Just as there are varying philosophical viewpoints in education, so, too, are there in speech-language pathology. We feel that communicative differences or disorders can affect the whole child: intellectual development, social development, psychological development, educational attainment, and future goals. Therefore, a speech-language pathologist is not responsible for merely treating a speech-language disorder but is also responsible for working with the whole child. In the same vein, teachers might ask themselves whether they teach reading or whether they teach children to read. The latter choice focuses on the child rather than on the behaviors to be taught. Furthermore, we believe that although there may be exceptions—notably the beginning stutterer—the majority of school-age children (and their parents) should know why they go to therapy. They should have some understanding of (1) their short-term and long-term goals (in general the child will be striving to achieve a new speech or language behavior and to make that behavior a habit), (2) how they will attempt to achieve these goals, (3) what the criteria are for goal achievement, and (4) why it is important to make changes or improvements in the way they communicate; in other words, they need to be motivated.

Scheduling

A schedule is a way of effectively and efficiently planning the use of time and of letting others know what will be (or is) going on at any particular time. A speech-language pathologist may serve one or many schools. One of the writers of this text has served as many as seven schools at a time. Needless to say, travel between schools can consume considerable time, especially when schools are far apart or if travel must occur near noon when traffic is heavier. The number of schools that can be served will vary with the following factors:

- The Size of Each School: It would be expected that the larger the school, the larger the number of students in need of therapy.
- The Time Required for Travel: The more time spent traveling, the less time is available for providing services.
- Other Duties and Responsibilities: If the speech-language pathologist is involved in district-wide assessment throughout the year, there will be less time available for providing services to individual schools.
- The Type of Program: In general, more students can be served within a given amount of time via collaborative consultation and monitoring programs than when pullout or community-based programs are provided. Obviously, only one school and a limited number of students would be served if the speech-language pathologist works with children in a self-contained program.

The speech-language pathologist should have at least one half-day, and in some school districts has a full day, of coordination time, when regularly sched-uled services are not provided, for such activities as assessment (both screening and individual evaluation); consultation with parents, teachers, and others; prepa-ration for and attendance at IEP conferences; paperwork; and preparation of ther-apy plans for the next week.

Prior to the passage of PL 94-142, most public school speech-language pathol-ogists had a list of students being served and a list of students waiting to be served. Now, in order to comply with federal law, there can be no waiting list (Healey & Dublinske, 1978). Each fall the speech-language pathologist identifies students and preschoolers with IEPs and IFSPs; notes individual time requirements per the IEPs and IFSPs for each child; and constructs a new schedule of children, times, and schools. Generally the speech-language pathologist will utilize more than one type of program to deliver the necessary and most appropriate services to various students. Schedules are not easy to complete and can be a potential source of controversy. Therefore, if a teacher has a request concerning the schedule, it is extremely helpful if that request is made to the speech-language pathologist as soon as possible and *before* the schedule is completed. Otherwise, to accommodate a change for one teacher, the speech-language pathologist must change another teacher's schedule, who may in turn dislike the new schedule. This does *not* mean, however, that a schedule will not change during the school year; schedules must be flexible. As a schedule changes, the therapy times of students in a particular class may be affected. Changes will occur as students are dismissed from therapy, newly identified and assessed children with completed IEPs or IFSPs are placed into therapy, and children are changed from one type of service delivery to another. For example, as a child improves, the duration or frequency of therapy may be decreased; if satisfactory progress does not occur, the duration or frequency may be increased. The original schedule and each new schedule will be distributed to the teachers. The complete schedule should be available in the principal's office in case a teacher needs to contact the speech-language pathologist at other school buildings.

There is also the question of just how many students with communication handicaps a speech-language pathologist should be responsible for at any one time. ASHA recommends a maximum caseload of 40 children and that that number should be reduced depending on the time requirements included in the IEPs and IFSPs (Guidelines for Caseload Size and Speech-Language Service Delivery in the Schools, 1993).

Will the Children in Need of Speech Therapy from a Single Classroom Go to Therapy at the Same Time?

Assuming that the children are involved in a program that takes them outside of the classroom, it is possible but not probable. In a pullout program some children will be seen individually and some will be seen in small groups, depending on their needs. The IEP will note whether therapy is individual and/or group. A child might even be seen both individually and in a small group each week. Group work may be especially appropriate because a social situation with peers can be simulated. The majority of speech-language pathologists group children homogeneously; that is, all the children in a group work on the same problem, such as stuttering or the "s" sound. A few speech-language pathologists group heterogeneously, grouping children together who are working on different types of problems; then it is more likely that children in a classroom will all be scheduled for therapy at the same time.

Consultation and Collaboration

Consultation is a process that "involves the interaction between two or more professionals for the purpose of mutually preventing or solving problems" (Heron &

Harris, 1982, p. 1). Some school professionals have a consultant's role as their primary job responsibility. However, in the context of this book, the consultation process occurs as just one responsibility of the speech-language pathologist and any other person who can bring to bear information, ideas, and techniques that can potentially and positively affect the communicative status of the child in question. The other person could be the regular classroom teacher, a special education teacher, a resource room teacher, a physical education teacher, a music teacher, an art teacher, a school nurse, a school psychologist, a counselor, the principal, a parent, or any other community resource personnel. The reader is right in interpreting this as an appeal for all concerned to think in terms of an interdisciplinary approach. The participants need to learn what each can contribute. It is of paramount importance that this team process be two-way, a give and take of information and ideas. Consider the following as examples of some of the possible interactions in which the speech-language pathologist might be involved.

Interactions with Parents

Contact with parents is mandatory as the approval for individual evaluation is obtained and as the IEP or IFSP is completed, but this should only be the first of a series of contacts during the year. Parents may be able to help reinforce at home the various achievements that have been made in therapy. They may also be able to provide information about how the child performs communicatively outside the school environment. During parental counseling, McFarlane, Fujiki, and Brinton (1984) suggest that the parents be encouraged to accept their child. They should be helped to understand that their child's communicative problem does not reflect on their value as parents or on the child, who needs just as much love and acceptance as any other child.

Interactions with the Classroom Teacher

The speech-language pathologist and teacher need to consult and collaborate with each other about the goals for a child, how they expect to accomplish these goals, and what success has been achieved. This can be accomplished formally or informally. It is helpful for the speech-language pathologist to provide the teacher with copies of written speech therapy progress reports that are sent home to the parents at grade reporting time.

Collaboration occurs more in some of the service delivery models and less in others. By definition, it occurs maximally in the classroom-based model. Much has been written about collaboration in both education and speech-language pathology literature. The bare-bones consensus is that all members of a collaboration team need to respect each other's areas of expertise; no one should feel intimidated or fear being judged by a teammate; and it requires time and commitment, administrative support in terms of providing the necessary time, and a blending of philosophies, work styles, and attitudes.

Collaboration can also consist of other knowledge sharing. For example, the classroom teacher usually has more contact with parents and spends more school hours with a child, who may talk about his or her feelings, wants, and life at home. Some information that a teacher receives from a child or parents may be important to the speech-language pathologist. For example, if parents complain that they still cannot understand a child who has shown such remarkable gains in intelligibility that the speech-language pathologist, teacher, and classmates now have little concern about intelligibility, the speech-language pathologist may want and need to discuss this matter with the parents. As another example, suppose that a teacher has as a student a stutterer, who was in therapy and had learned to control the stuttering except occasionally in stressful situations. If the teacher is informed of stressful situations at home, especially if the situation will be of some duration, like a separation or divorce of the parents, and informs the speech-language pathologist, the speech-language pathologist with the parents' permission may confer with the student and review strategies for controlling the stuttering. In this way, increased stuttering may be averted or at least minimized. The stutterer may also be reminded to contact the speech-language pathologist for help at any time.

The teacher is also in a position to provide the speech-language pathologist with information about a child's speech and language skills in the classroom and in informal situations, such as in the hallway, in the lunchroom, or on the playground. The teacher can also provide reminders to the child during the habit-forming stages of therapy, when the child can produce the targeted speech behaviors but still must make them a habit in all communicative situations. As noted earlier in this chapter, this stage of therapy is referred to as "carryover."

In return, the speech-language pathologist can serve as a resource for the teacher, as the speech-language pathologist may have more experience with language disorders or methods for promoting phonological readiness and auditory-visual skills necessary for reading. Specifically, the speech-language pathologist may provide and even demonstrate activities for the teachers, such as ways to develop auditory-verbal skills. This ability to act as a resource is, in essence, the premise that the indirect collaborative consultation therapy program is based on.

Another example of consultation between the classroom teacher and speech-language pathologist involves the use of classroom materials as a source for therapeutic materials. This may be more appropriate at some stages of therapy than at others. However, especially for students experiencing learning difficulties, this could provide more exposure to classroom material in a somewhat different environment. Once the speech-language pathologist and classroom teacher have developed a working relationship, the time spent in communicating about use of appropriate classroom materials in the therapy situation should be minimal and could certainly be worthwhile. The carryover stage of therapy provides many possibilities for reinforcement of classroom materials. For example, a child with a distorted "r" sound might read a portion of a lesson to the speech-language pathologist while practicing a correctly produced "r" sound. A group of children working to establish a correctly produced "s" or working to eliminate the hoarse quality in their voices might discuss a social studies unit with the speech-language pathologist. This could provide the students with an opportunity to determine which sections of the unit each especially needs to review for an upcoming test. Fellows (1976) suggested that utilization of classroom materials works even at the secondary level, giving as examples the use of textbook glossaries or a drivers' education manual for therapeutic materials.

Interactions with Other School Personnel

The physical education teacher, the art teacher, the principal, the office secretary, and others can learn from the speech-language pathologist what to do when a stutterer stutters or how to better and more easily communicate with a hearing-impaired child. The speech-language pathologist can utilize the information provided by other school personnel while contributing to that other professional's work. For example, the psychologist and speech-language pathologist might discuss how the results of speech and language tests can be interpreted with respect to the psychologist's findings of cognitive and emotional status or how intelligence tests that rely heavily on linguistic ability should be interpreted for the child who is language impaired. Just as in the case of the classroom teacher, the speech-language pathologist and resource room teachers also need to consult in order to appropriately help a child. For example, because expressive and receptive verbal abilities are prerequisite to learning to read, the speech-language pathologist and reading specialist may both work with some of the same children and will need to communicate and coordinate their goals, techniques, and materials.

Community Resource

The speech-language pathologist may also utilize community resources in providing the best services. The otolaryngologist's report about the physical status of the vocal folds of a child with a hoarse, breathy voice will determine whether or not that child is an appropriate candidate for voice therapy. For the child with an unusual problem the speech-language pathologist might want a second opinion. A nearby university speech, language, and hearing clinic might be an ideal place to obtain more information or a second opinion. The speech-language pathologist may initiate referrals for therapy during the summer months. This might involve therapy at local resources or at camps specializing in various speech problems, such as the Shady Trails Camp, associated with the University of Michigan, which incorporates speech therapy into a traditional summer camp. The speech-language pathologist may maintain contacts with state and local agencies and with community philanthropic organizations that might provide financial assistance for adaptive communication devices (discussed in Chapter 8).

Summary

Some Important Points to Remember

- All teachers can expect to have children with communicative disorders in their classrooms.

- The emotional and social adjustments of children as well as their educational achievement are related to communication skills.
- The speech-language pathologist is the professional who is prepared to work with children having communicative problems.
- The American Speech-Language-Hearing Association is the professional organization that sets standards for speech-language pathologists and audiologists.
- The audiologist is concerned with hearing and hearing disorders and their remediation.
- The Individuals with Disabilities Education Act (IDEA) and its amendments address the educational needs of children with disabilities by stressing inclusion.
- An Individualized Educational Program (IEP) must be completed for each handicapped school-age child, and the education must be provided in the least restrictive environment (LRE).
- The IEP is drawn up by a team of school personnel and the child's parent(s).
- An Individualized Family Service Plan (IFSP) focuses on both the preschooler and the child's family.
- Communicative disorders are among the most prevalent handicapping conditions in the United States.
- The term *communication* implies a transfer of ideas, opinions, and feelings via *language*, which is a formalized system by which we communicate.
- *Speech* is the spoken production of language.
- The components of language include: (1) syntax, (2) semantics, (3) morphology, (4) pragmatics, and (5) phonology.
- Seven types of service delivery programs for children in the public schools are: monitoring, collaborative consultation, classroom-based, pullout, self-contained, community-based, and combination.
- The responsibilities of the speech-language pathologist involve: (1) assessment, (2) therapy, (3) scheduling, and (4) consultation and collaboration.
- Teachers should discuss observing speech therapy sessions with the speech-language pathologist.
- Speech-language pathologists are interested in the total development of a child's communicative skills.
- It is important that children and parents understand why the child is in therapy.
- The scheduling of therapy for any child must be jointly accomplished by the teacher and the speech-language pathologist.
- Generally the speech-language pathologist serves more than one school building.
- If more than one child from a classroom receives therapy, they might not all leave and return to the room together—this depends on the nature of the disorders.
- The speech-language pathologist frequently confers with teachers, other professionals, and parents.

Self-Test

Fill in the Blank:

1. Otitis media is _____.

2. The problem with the various forms of otitis media is that they may cause _____.

3. The purpose of screening is to _____.

4. IEP stands for _____.

5. LRE stands for _____.

6. Inclusion refers to children with disabilities being included in the regular _____ and the regular _____.

7. The seven service delivery models discussed are _____, _____, _____, _____, _____, _____, and _____.

8. The ability to produce a sound with or without specific directions is referred to as _____.

9. The five dimensions of language are _____, _____, _____, _____, and _____.

10. Work with other professionals to prevent or solve problems has been referred to as _____.

True or False:

1. The various services, including speech therapy, that a child may receive depend on the disability category within which a child falls. _____

2. Regular education teachers seldom are part of an IEP committee. _____

3. Reading and writing are examples of expressive language. _____

4. A communicative disorder exists when the listener pays more attention to how the message is communicated than to what is being communicated. _____

5. The cause of the communicative disorder must be determined before therapy is initiated. _____

6. Parents must give permission for their children to be screened for communicative problems. _____

7. Kindergartners are always screened for communicative problems. _____

8. Secondary teachers do not need to be concerned with making referrals to the speech-language pathologist. _____

9. Children on a waiting list will receive speech therapy just as soon as there is an opening in the speech-language pathologist's schedule. _____

10. Speech, language, and hearing services for articulation problems, such as a ———
"w" substitution for an "r," may be considered special education under
federal law.

References

Ad Hoc Committee on the Roles and Responsibilities of the School-Based Speech-Language Pathologist (1999). *Guidelines for the roles and responsibilities of the school-based speech-language pathologist.* Rockville, MD: American Speech-Language-Hearing Association.

Amiot, A. (1998). Policy, politics, and the power of information: The critical need for outcomes and clinical trials data in policy-making in the schools. *ASHA, 29,* 245.

Baum, H. M. (1998). Overview, definitions, and goals for ASHA's treatment outcomes and clinical trials activities (What difference do outcome data make to you?). *ASHA, 29,* 246–249.

Blosser, J. L., & Kratcoski, A. (1997). PACs: A framework for determining appropriate service delivery options. *ASHA, 28,* 99–107.

Bolton, W. F. (1981). Language: An introduction. In V. P. Clark, P. A. Eschholz, & A. F. Rosa (Eds.), *Language* (3rd ed.) (pp. 1–17). New York: St. Martin's Press.

Coleman, T. J., Thompson-Smith, T., Pruitt, G. D., & Richards, L. N. (1999). Rural service delivery: Unique challenges, creative solutions. *ASHA, 41*(1), 40–45.

Davolt, S. (1999a). Clinton proposes $4 million for newborn hearing screening. *ASHA Leader* 4(5), 1–2.

Davolt, S. (1999b). Universal infant hearing screening gains momentum in states. *ASHA Leader* 4(8), 1, 5.

Elksnin, L. K., & Capilouto, G. J. (1994). Speech-language pathologists: Perceptions of integrated service delivery in school settings. *Language, Speech, and Hearing Services in Schools, 25,* 258–267.

English, K., & Church, G. (1999). Unilateral hearing loss in children: An update for the 1990s. *ASHA, 30,* 26–31.

Farber, J. G., & Klein, E. R. (1999). Classroom-based assessment of a collaborative intervention program with kindergarten and first-grade students. *ASHA, 30*(1) 83–91.

Fellows, J. B. (1976). The speech pathologist in the high school setting. *Language, Speech, and Hearing Services in Schools, 7,* 61–63.

Gallagher, T. M., Swigert, N. B, & Baum, H. M. (1998). Collecting outcomes data in schools: Needs and challenges. *ASHA, 29,* 270–273.

Gantwerk, B. (1985). Assessment issues in decision making. In *Caseload issues in schools* (pp. 25–34). Rockville, MD: American Speech-Language-Hearing Association.

Guidelines for caseload size and speech-language service delivery in the schools (1993). *ASHA, 35,* suppl. 10, 33–39.

Guidelines for caseload size for speech-language services in the schools (1984). *ASHA, 26*(4), 53–58.

Healey, W. C., & Dublinske, S. (1978). Notes from the school services program. *Language, Speech, and Hearing Services in Schools, 9,* 203.

Heron, T. E., & Harris, K. C. (1982). *The educational consultant: Helping professionals, parents and mainstreamed students.* Boston: Allyn & Bacon.

Janota, J. (1999). Otitis media (1999). *ASHA, 41*(1), 48.

Job opportunities ahead for speech-language pathologists, audiologists. (1998). *ASHA Leader, 3*(19), 6

Karr, S. (1999). Action: School services. *Language, Speech, and Hearing Services in Schools, 30,* 212–220.

Logemann, J. A. (1998). Treatment outcomes and efficacy in the schools. *ASHA, 29,* 243–244.

Matthews, J. (1986). The professions of speech-language pathology and audiology. In G. H. Shames & E. H. Wigg (Eds.), *Human communication disorders* (2nd ed.) (pp. 3–26). Columbus, OH: Merrill.

McDermott, L. (1985). Service alternatives. In *Caseload issues in schools* (pp. 18–24). Rockville,

MD: American Speech-Language-Hearing Association.

McFarlane, S. C., Fujiki, M., & Brinton, B. (1984). *Coping with communication handicaps.* San Diego, CA: College-Hill.

Montgomery, J. K., & Fujikawa, S. (1992). Hearing thresholds of students in the second, eighth, and twelfth grades. *Language, Speech, and Hearing Services in Schools, 23,* 61–63.

Moore, P., & Kester, D. C. (1953). Historical notes in speech correction in the pre-association era. *Journal of Speech and Hearing Disorders, 18,* 48–53.

Neal, W. R., Jr. (1976). Speech pathology services in the secondary schools. *Language, Speech, and Hearing Services in Schools, 7,* 6–16.

New bill supports early identification of hearing loss (1999). *ASHA Leader, 4*(6), 1.

New proposed AuD standards published (1997). *ASHA Leader, 2*(13), 1, 8–9.

Number of students with disabilities rises (1995). *ASHA, 37*(1), 14.

Ohio Board of Speech Language Pathology and Audiology (1997). *Ohio Law and Rules Governing Speech-Language Pathology and Audiology Aides,* Section 4753.072.

Peters-Johnson, C. (1996). ASHA completes national schools survey. *Language, Speech, and Hearing Services in Schools, 27,* 185–186.

Peters-Johnson, C. (1997). Action: School services—Fast facts from 1995 ASHA school survey. *Language, Speech, and Hearing Services in Schools, 28,* 91–93.

Peters-Johnson, C. (1998). Action: School services. *Language, Speech, and Hearing Services in Schools, 29,* 186–190.

Phillips, P. P. (1976). Variables affecting classroom teachers' understanding of speech disorders. *Language, Speech, and Hearing Services in Schools, 7,* 142–149.

Porterfield K. (1998). British researchers identify genetic area affecting speech. *ASHA Leader 3*(4), 1, 4.

Research conference highlights advances in genetics research (1996). *ASHA Leader, 1*(25), 10.

Roberts, J. E., & Medley, L. P. (1995). Otitis media and speech-language sequelae in young children: Current issues in management. *American Journal of Speech-Language Pathology, 4,* 15–24.

Ross, M. (1994). Overview of aural rehabilitation. In J. Katz (Ed.), *Handbook of clinical audiology* (4th ed.) (pp. 587–596). Baltimore, MD: Williams & Wilkins.

School services: Answers to frequently asked questions (1998). Rockville, MD: American Speech-Language-Hearing Association.

Seymour, C. M. (1997). Research, graduate education, and the future of our professions. *ASHA, 39*(3), 7.

Task force report on school speech, hearing, and language screening procedures (1973). *Language, Speech, and Hearing Services in Schools, 4,* 109–119.

Uffen, E. (1997). Speech and language disorders: Nature or nurture? *ASHA Leader, 2*(14), 8.

Van Riper, C., & Emerick, L. (1984). *Speech correction: An introduction to speech pathology and audiology.* Englewood Cliffs, NJ: Prentice-Hall.

Who has hearing, speech, and language problems? (1995). *ASHA, 37*(2), 38–39.

Work, R. S. (1985). The therapy program. In R. J. Van Hattum (Ed.), *Organization of speech-language services in schools* (pp. 286–337). San Diego, CA: College-Hill.

C h a p t e r 2

Articulation and Phonological Disorders

It is probably safe to make two wagers. The first is that everyone reading this book has heard a young child make errors in speech sound production. The child may have called a rabbit a "wabbit" or said "Mith Thmith" instead of "Miss Smith." In the first instance a "w" sound was substituted for an "r" sound, and in the second instance a "th" sound was substituted for an "s" sound. Both of these are very typical errors. The second wager is that the reader has also heard an adult make speech sound errors. Possibly the "s" sound was distorted, sounding either slushy and indistinct or as though it were combined with a noisy whistle. Some speakers are able to overcome the negative impressions that such errors create through strong personal assets. However, other speakers who make speech sound errors are thought to be less intelligent, less well educated, less physically attractive, or less socially attractive (Crowe-Hall, 1991; Mowrer, 1974, cited in Shriberg, 1980; Mowrer, Wahl, & Doolan, 1978; Perrin, 1954; Silverman, 1976, 1986; Silverman & Falk, 1992; Silverman & Paulus, 1989). Children and adults exhibiting such errors are often called names, teased, or laughed at. Children (and unfortunately even adults) sometimes make fun of a person with speech sound problems by mimicking that individual's speech.

What Is a Speech Sound?

A speech sound is generally called a *phoneme* by speech-language pathologists. Technically, it is the smallest sound segment in a word that we can hear and that, when changed, modifies the meaning of a word. For example, the words "bit" and "bid" have different meanings yet differ in their respective sounds by only the last sound of each word (i.e., "t" and "d"). These two sounds are phonemes because

29

they are capable of changing meaning. Speech sounds or phonemes are classified as vowels and consonants. In English, as most readers are aware, the letters of a word and the sounds of a word do not always have a one-to-one correspondence. This will be clearer with an example. Consider the word "squirrel." It has eight letters but only five sounds: "s"–"k"–"w"–"r"–"l."

To avoid some of this confusion, speech-language pathologists use symbols from the International Phonetic Alphabet (IPA) to represent each speech sound. Many of these IPA symbols, which are enclosed in slashes or brackets depending on how the symbol is used, are the same as the letters we use, but some are not. However, rather than ask you to learn these symbols, in this book the letters in the alphabet enclosed in quotation marks, such as "s," will be used to represent the various speech sounds as they are discussed. In order to do this, some letters will need additional information attached to them for clarity. For example, to represent the first sound in "jam" the phrase "j as in jam" will be used. (See Table 2-2 and the section on consonants.)

Vowel and Diphthongs

The vowels and diphthongs (a *diphthong* is the sound that results when the articulators move from one vowel to another within the same syllable) used in American English are listed in Table 2-1. Each one of these vowels and diphthongs is a speech sound or phoneme. When asked how many vowels there are in the alphabet, the answer may be a, e, i, o, u, and sometimes y, but when referring to speech, the number of vowels increases. In other words, there are five or six vowel letters but approximately 17 distinct vowel sounds. (Remember that there are some variations in vowel usage due to regional or dialectical differences.)

Consonants

The consonants in English and the way they will be referred to are listed in Table 2-2. Speech-language pathologists, speech scientists, linguists, and others interested in speech and language frequently describe consonants by their place of articulation and manner of articulation as well as the presence or absence of voicing. Table 2-3 provides such information. You should note from this table that many consonant sounds are produced alike, except for the voicing factor. For instance, "p" and

TABLE 2-1   The Vowels and Diphthongs in English (the italicized portions)

h*ea*t	w*ou*ld	h*ai*l
h*i*t	h*u*t	b*oi*l
h*a*t	*a*bout	h*ow*
h*ea*d	*a*ll	h*ur*t
h*o*t	h*o*pe	lett*er*
f*oo*d	h*igh*	

TABLE 2-2   The Consonant Sounds in English

Symbol Used in This Book		Examples	
"p"	pig	apple	cup
"b"	bus	ribbon	crib
"t"	toy	button	light
"d"	dime	ladder	red
"k"	choir	bouquet	duck
"g"	ghost	buggy	egg
"m"	monkey	hammer	comb
"n"	knee	tennis	bacon
"ng"		finger	ring
"voiceless th"	thumb	toothpaste	teeth
"voiced th"	this	feather	smooth
"f"	foot	buffalo	graph
"v"	vacuum	seven	five
"s"	scene	bicycle	grass
"z"	zoo	puzzle	dogs
"sh"	sugar	ocean	moustache
"zh"		television	mirage
"ch"	cello	question	match
"j as in jam"	jet	soldier	badge
"l"	lion	pillow	ball
"r"	rhyme	carrot	car
"w"	watch	towel	
"hw"	white		
"h"	house	tomahawk	
"y as in yo-yo"	yarn	onion	

"b" are both bilabial (made with both lips) stops (the flow of air in the vocal tract is completely stopped and then released at the place of articulation). However, one is produced with voicing (the vocal folds are vibrating) and the other is produced without voicing (the vocal folds are not vibrating). The terms *voiced* and *voiceless* are used to refer to the presence or absence of voicing. When voicing is the only difference in sound production between two sounds, they are referred to as *cognates*. Frequently, when children have difficulty producing one sound of a cognate pair, they also have difficulty with the other sound in the pair. Thus, if they are enrolled in therapy, they will work on both sounds. Note that when uttering a consonant sound, one should not attach a vowel to that sound. For example, the "s" sound says only "s" not "es" and "t" is not "tee" or "tuh."

What Types of Speech Sound Problems Do Children Exhibit?

Errors may be of the following types:

1. Distortions: A speech sound or phoneme is said to be distorted when it sounds more like the intended sound than any other speech sound yet is noticeably

TABLE 2-3   Speech Sounds in English Described by Their Place of Articulation, Manner of Articulation, and the Presence or Absence of Voicing

Manner of Articulation		Place of Articulation						
		Bilabial	Labiodental	Linguadental	Alveolar	Palatal	Velar	Glottal
Stops	VL	p			t		k	
	V	b			d		g	
Fricatives	VL		f	th	s	sh		h
	V		v	th	z	zh		
Affricates	VL					ch		
	V					j as in jam		
Nasals	V	m			n		ng	
Liquids	V				l	r		
Glides	VL	hw						
	V	w				y as in yo-yo		

Place of articulation refers to the location of the constriction that occurs as the consonant is produced: Bilabial—both lips, Labiodental—the lower lip and upper front teeth, Linguadental—the tip of the tongue between the front teeth, Alveolar—the tongue and the ridge behind the teeth, Palatal—the tongue and the hard palate, Velar—the tongue and the soft palate (velum), Glottal—the space between the vocal folds.

Manner of articulation refers to the manner of release and/or the type of constriction within the vocal tract: Stops—sounds produced when airflow is momentarily blocked (stopped) at the place of articulation, Fricatives—sounds produced when airflow is reduced (causing friction) at the place of articulation, Affricates—sounds produced when airflow is first blocked and then constricted, Nasals—sounds produced when airflow behind the constriction is directed through the nose rather than through the mouth, Liquids—sounds that are vowel-like but not produced with an open vocal tract, Glides—sounds produced by the movement of the articulators from one position to another and that occur before vowels or diphthongs.
VL = voiceless, V = voiced.

wrong. Example: The "r" in "reading" is produced so that it sounds strange but is more like an "r" than any other speech sound.

2. Substitutions: A substitution occurs when one speech sound is substituted for another. Example: "f" is substituted for "voiceless th" when a child announces that he has hurt his "fum" instead of his "thumb."

3. Omissions: An omission occurs when a speech sound is simply left out. Example: The "r" is omitted when a child counts to "fo" instead of "four."

4. Additions: An addition occurs when a speech sound that does not belong, and is not replacing another sound, is added to a word. Example: A child may insert the unstressed vowel that occurs in the first syllable of "*about*" into the color "blue" between the *b* and *l*, thus saying "buhlue." You should be aware that this type of error can occur, but because it occurs infrequently in the school-age population, it will not be discussed any further in this chapter.

Any child may exhibit a combination of errors (distortions, substitutions, and omissions) across sounds or on any one sound. For example, a child may distort one pair of sounds, such as the "sh" and "zh," and exhibit substitution errors on another pair of sounds, such as "voiceless th" for "s" and "voiced th" for "z." For example, this child would distort "zh" in television, distort "sh" in she, say "bathket" for "basket," and say "thithorth" for "scissors." Yet another child may substitute "w" or the vowel in "would" for "l" in initial and medial positions and may omit "l" in final positions and in *blends* (a blend consists of two or more consecutive consonants in the same syllable, such as *bl*end or *str*ipe), so that more than one type of error is produced for an individual sound. This child would say "wesson" instead of "lesson,", "sawad" for "salad," "ba" for "ball," and "fashwight" for "flashlight."

Sometimes speech sound errors cause the meaning of the intended word to be changed, so that unless the listener can determine from the context what the intended word is, *intelligibility* (how easily listeners can understand what a speaker is saying) is decreased. Imagine a teacher's momentary confusion when, on the first day of school, a child announces, "My daddy is a coat." The child, who substitutes "t" for "ch," was really intending to say, "My daddy is a coach." A teacher may not fare much better in understanding a child who, out of the blue, asks, "Do you see?" However, if this question was asked in the context of a discussion about the first big snowfall, a teacher would probably be quick to catch on to the fact that the question refers to skiing. Although the child could produce "s" correctly, she could not produce the "sk" blend in the word "ski." Another child may sound as if he is asking "Is this white?" when he means "Is this right?" A "w" for "r" substitution occurred in the initial position of the word "right." A teacher might respond, "Tear what?" to a child complaining, "He won't tear," when really the child is trying to say, "He won't share."

Intelligibility is affected by the type of error. Distortions are the most easily understood, followed by substitutions, and then omissions, which are considered the most immature sounding of these errors. Common substitutions, such as "voiceless th" for "s," "voiced th" for "z," "w" for "r," "w" for "l," and "f" or "t" for "voiceless th," are easier to understand than unusual substitutions, such as "l" for "r." For example, the statement "We glow loses" would be more difficult to understand than "We gwow woses" for "We grow roses."

The number of errors made is also related to intelligibility. Think about the child who has many such errors in speech. Such a child might say "Aah nie mama n I hah tuh geh my ih . . uh . a new aah . . ke . cau umbah . . ee tol huh ol one" for "Last night Mama and I had to get my sister a new jacket because somebody stole her old one" (periods are used to indicate a degree of prolongation of the preceding sound). A stranger, or someone who has no idea what the child might be talking about, may find this communication unintelligible. Compare this to "At retheth today, can Tharah and I go outthide of the fenth to pick thome flowerth?" for "At recess today, can Sarah and I go outside of the fence to pick some flowers?" Even though there are many errors in this request, all errors are consistent substitutions occurring on "s" or "z" sounds. A stranger might have to listen closely but should be able to understand what the child is saying.

Children should be intelligible to strangers by the time they are 3 to 4 years old (Shriberg, 1980). That does not mean that they have no errors in their speech;

it simply means that they can be understood fairly easily. In fact, it has been estimated (Pendergast, 1966) that one-fourth of the first-grade population misarticulates one or more speech sounds. Teachers who work with younger children (preschoolers, kindergartners, and first-graders) are the ones most likely to deal with children whose speech is sometimes unintelligible. Even parents report that they do not always understand what their child says. If listeners can contextually narrow a child's message by asking the child to point to what he or she is referring to, or by asking questions that can be answered with one-word responses, they are more apt to be able to understand what the child is trying to say.

Traditionally all speech sound errors were labeled as problems in articulation and were considered to be relatively simple (McReynolds, 1986). However, since the late 1970s, research has demonstrated that speech sound errors are more complex than previously thought, thus causing changes in how errors are classified. New classifications include errors of articulation and errors of phonology. The reader will first be introduced to articulatory disorders and then to phonological disorders. Sections on assessment and treatment of both types of disorders will follow.

Articulation

What Is Articulation?

Articulation refers to the actual movements of the speech organs that occur during the production of various speech sounds. Successful articulation requires (1) neurological integrity; (2) normal respiration; (3) normal action of the larynx (voice box or Adam's apple); (4) normal movement of the articulators, which include the tongue, teeth, hard palate, soft palate, lips, and mandible (lower jaw); and (5) adequate hearing.

When Should a Child No Longer Have Articulatory Errors?

In other words, by what age should a child achieve the accepted "adult" standard of articulation? Research has shown that there tends to be a natural developmental sequence to speech sound acquisition and that it is reasonable to expect different sounds to be learned at different ages. Most researchers have agreed on which sounds are learned earlier and which are learned later. The primary differences have been in the exact ages that are associated with the acquisition of each sound. Many of these differences have been related to how ages were calculated (e.g., the age at which 75 percent of the children in a study had acquired the sound in all word positions versus the age at which 50 percent of the children had acquired the sound in two out of three word positions). If a child has not yet reached the age at which the sound should be learned, the sound error is considered to be a *maturational* or *developmental articulation error*. A teacher should accept such errors as a normal part of childhood.

Although most data are reported by age, the following guidelines are presented by grade level because it should be easier for the teacher to remember and use as a basis for referral to the speech-language pathologist. Remember that this information is a "rule of thumb"; the speech-language pathologist will also be looking at the child's exact age as well as other factors.

By kindergarten age:	"p," "b," "m," "n," "h," "w," "t," "d," "k," "g," "ng," "f," "y as in yo-yo"
By first grade:	"l"
By second grade:	"ch," "sh," "j as in jam"
By third grade:	"voiceless th," "voiced th," "r," "s," "z," "v," "zh"

Some schools will use acquisition data showing slightly later ages/grades, especially for the "s," "z," and "r," pushing them up to "by fourth grade." Whatever age or grade has been used, once it is reached, it is assumed that maturation will no longer play a role in the child's acquisition of that particular sound. A child would then be eligible to work in therapy on that sound. (Remember, though, that the IEP committee makes the final decision.)

According to Shriberg (1980), vowel acquisition is normally expected by 3 to 4 years of age. The exception to this is when the stressed and unstressed "er" sounds (as in "hurt" and "letter") are classified as vowels versus syllabic consonants, as these sounds will be acquired about the same time as the consonantal "r." The remaining vowels will not be discussed any further in this chapter, because the majority of children will have mastered them by school age. However, it should be noted that school-age bilingual children and children with organic problems, such as cerebral palsy, cleft palate, and hearing impairments, may have difficulty articulating vowels as well as difficulty with consonants. This will be referred to again in appropriate chapters.

Teachers may be asked to use a consonant acquisition chart or guideline for determining how concerned they should be about a child's articulation and whether or not they should make a referral to a speech-language pathologist. For example, according to the preceding information, a child in second grade who continues to have articulation errors on the "l" sound should be referred to a speech-language pathologist. However, a kindergarten or first-grade child who substitutes the "th" sounds for the "s" and "z" sounds would fall well within the maturational time span for these sounds. These errors would be considered typical for the age, and a teacher might rightfully choose not to refer this child to a speech-language pathologist for testing. However, a word of caution: Teachers should not rely on such a guideline exclusively. For example, a first-grader could correctly produce all sounds corresponding to his grade level and could err on all other sounds, which means that 10 sounds would be misarticulated. Such a child would be difficult to understand at times, if not unintelligible. This child should be referred. In fact, any child who is difficult to understand should be referred to a speech-language pathologist, regardless of any guidelines to the contrary.

What Sounds Are School-Age Children Most Apt to Have Difficulty With?

Speech-language pathologists working in schools indicate that the most frequently misarticulated sounds are "r" (including the syllabic consonant "er") and "s" (along with its cognate "z"). In fact, it has been reported that errors on the "r" and "s" sounds are the most common errors made in speech by both children and adults (Shriberg, 1980). Typical errors on "r" include substituting a "w" or the vowel in "would" for "r" and distorting the "r." Various substitutions, notably "voiceless th" for "s," "voiced th" for "z," and sometimes "t" for "s" and "d" for "z," occur along with distorted "s" and "z" sounds. The "voiceless th" and "voiced th" substitutions for "s" and "z" are frequently referred to as a *frontal lisp.* The term *lateral lisp* is sometimes used to refer to distorted "s," "z," "ch," "j as in jam," "sh," and "zh" sounds. Producing this slushy sound can be approximated by attempting to say "s" while the tongue is in the position for an "l" sound (Shriberg, 1980). Try it, and feel how air is emitted on either side of the tongue (laterally) rather than down the center of the tongue. Other commonly misarticulated sounds in the school-age population include "l," "ch," "j as in jam," "sh," "voiced th," and "voiceless th." Young children who are unintelligible are also likely to exhibit errors on "k," "g," and "f."

Churchill, Hodson, Jones, and Novak (1988) found that children between the approximate ages of 4 and 6 with histories of recurrent otitis media during their first 2 years had a higher incidence of "s" errors than did children without histories of recurrent otitis media. They hypothesized that the "s" errors could be accounted for by early hearing loss associated with otitis media.

Phonology

Phonology is one component of language. A broader concept than articulation, *phonology* involves the study of speech sounds and the rule system for combining speech sounds into meaningful words. Children must perceive and produce speech sounds and acquire the rules of the language used in their environment. Some familiar rules involve permissible sequences of speech sounds. For example, in American English a blend of two consonants such as s and t is permissible at the beginning of a word but blending the two consonants k and b is not; ng is not produced at the beginning of words; and w is not produced at the end of words (words may end in the letter w but not the sound "w"). Marketing experts demonstrate their knowledge of phonology when they coin words for new products; product names chosen are recognizable to the public as rightful words. Slang also follows these rules. For example, consider the word "nerd." It is recognizable as an acceptably formed noun. Game lovers demonstrate such knowledge when they play Hangman. Given a word in which the next to the last letter is r, they know that some letter combinations, such as rh at the end of a word would not be logical;

sequences, such as *ry, rn, rs,* or *re,* would be better guesses. Children acquire these underlying rules and principles as normal phonological development occurs.

As children experience normal phonological development, they may use certain phonological processes or rules to simplify adult forms of speech until they are capable of correct production. In other words, it is assumed that, for whatever reason, children naturally simplify adult forms that are difficult for them to produce at that point in their development (Ingram, 1976; Schwartz, 1983). The terms *phonological processes* and *phonological rules* have been coined to represent these simplifications (Edwards & Shriberg, 1983; Hodson, 1980, 1992; Ingram, 1976; Stoel-Gammon & Dunn, 1985). Each phonological process is applicable to several sounds at the same time. Examples of common phonological processes or rules include:

1. Deletion of final consonant (e.g., "ba" is used for "bat," "bath," "bad," "badge," and "back")
2. Deletion of unstressed syllable (e.g., "member" is used for "remember")
3. Cluster (blend) reduction (e.g., "tove" is used for "stove" and "wing" (with an age-appropriate substitution of "w" for "r") is used for "bring," "spring," and "string")
4. Various types of assimilation, in which one sound in a word affects another sound (e.g., "gog" is used for "dog" as the last sound in the word affects the first sound)
5. Fronting, in which sounds made in the back of the mouth are replaced by sounds made toward the front of the mouth (e.g., "bat" is used for "back" as the front sound "t" replaces the back sound "k")
6. Stopping, in which stops replace fricatives (see Table 2-3) (e.g., "tee" is used for "see" with the stop "t" replacing the fricative "s")

It should be noted that even though a child uses a particular phonological process, he or she probably does not use it 100 percent of the time. For example, a child will not omit *every* final consonant. Generally at least the "m," "n," and perhaps the easier consonants, such as "p" and "b," will be used in the final position.

Let's reemphasize that each phonological process is applicable to several sounds at the same time and use this fact as a basis to help distinguish an articulatory disorder from a phonological disorder. If a child omits one sound all of the time and even with a little help cannot say that sound, it is probably an articulatory disorder, and the child needs to be taught how to say that sound. However, if a child omits final consonants much of the time, yet says many of these sounds in the initial position of words (for example, "ca" is used for "cat" but "two" is said with a correct "t"), the problem is phonological. The child does not need to be taught to say "t" but does need to be taught the importance of saying all the word.

As children mature, these phonological processes should disappear and be replaced with the adult form of sound production. When such processes do not disappear and continue past the time that they should be eliminated, a child is said to have a phonological disorder. Haelsig and Madison (1986) found that the greatest decrease in the use of phonological processes occurred between 3 and 4 years of age. Interestingly this coincides with the age at which children are expected to be intelligible to strangers.

However, stop for a moment and think about the intelligibility of a child with a phonological disorder whose speech is characterized by more than one phonological rule or process (which may also be called a phonological deviation when continued to be used longer than it should be). Not an uncommon occurrence is the preschool child (or the kindergartner who has had no speech therapy) whose speech is characterized by final consonant deletion, fronting, stopping, and cluster reduction. This child says "t" plus long vowel "a" ("tay") for the following words: "say," letter *k*, "take," "cake," "cage," "Kate," "trade," "shade," "shake," "skate," and "face" along with many more possibilities.

What Causes Articulatory or Phonological Errors to Occur?

For young children, articulatory errors may represent a stage in the normal development of speech. However, when certain milestones have passed and a child continues to make certain errors, questions as to why should be formulated and answers sought. *Etiology* refers to the study of causes. Etiological factors can be considered to be either organic or functional.

Organic causes are ones that relate to structural or physiological abnormalities. These are identifiable causes, such as

- Hearing loss (see chapters 6 and 7)
- Cleft palate (see chapter 5)
- Missing or malformed oral structures
- Syndromes that may involve orofacial anomalies, mental handicaps, hearing loss, etc.
- Muscular problems such as paralysis or weakness
- Cerebral palsy (see chapter 8)
- Developmental dysarthria (a neurological problem)
- Childhood apraxia (difficulty with the motor planning and sequencing of speech in the absence of muscular difficulty)
- Other neurological problems

These might be related to hereditary factors, factors that occurred during pregnancy, birth trauma, accidents, or diseases. If possible, remediation (sometimes requiring a team of medical and related professionals) will directly address the organic problem. For example, surgery may correct a cleft palate. However, if an organic problem cannot be corrected, therapeutic goals and procedures must take into account the structural or physiological condition.

Causes are labeled *functional* when no apparent organic or physiological problem is present. Imitation of a poor speech model, little opportunity to speak, and faulty learning fall into this category. Often the word "functional" acts like a wastebasket term when a cause is simply unknown. Most speech sound problems are functional in nature; that is, no cause can be found and a child does indeed respond to therapy, learning to produce "normal" speech.

In their search for causes, researchers have investigated a wide variety of factors. Following is a list of some of these factors and a brief statement about each (Bernthal & Bankson, 1981; McReynolds, 1986; Shriberg, 1980; Webster & Plante, 1992).

- Intelligence: There appears to be little relationship between articulation and intelligence when intelligence falls within the normal range. However, children with intelligence quotients (IQs) below 70 will be more apt to have articulatory or phonological problems than those with IQs above 70. Therefore, special education teachers may expect a larger percentage of their children to exhibit speech sound errors and to possibly require speech therapy.
- Auditory Discrimination: There is evidence indicating a relationship, although it may not be causal, between auditory discrimination (the ability to discriminate between speech sounds) and the ability to correctly produce speech sounds.
- Phonological Awareness: Children who are moderately to severely unintelligible may have poorer phonological awareness abilities, e.g., awareness of language segments (number of words in a sentence, number of syllables in a word, and number of sounds in a word), than do children who are intelligible. Because of a relationship between phonological awareness and academic success, this is discussed later in this chapter.
- Gender: Some studies have indicated that at certain ages, girls have better speech sound production than boys, but few of these differences have been statistically significant.
- Dentition: Over all, there appears to be no consistent relationship between dentition problems, such as misaligned teeth or poor bite, and poor sound production. Certain types of lisps may be associated with poor dentition, but children have a capacity for compensating for poor dentition. Loss of baby teeth does not seem to affect the production of sounds that have already been learned because compensatory movements are quickly and unconsciously learned. Similarly, braces and other orthodontic appliances may temporarily interfere with clear articulation, but compensatory movements are quickly learned and used for the duration of the orthodontic treatment.
- Oral Structures: There does not seem to be a relationship between size and shape of the tongue, lips, or hard palate and speech sound production unless the abnormality is extreme. As with dentition, children appear to be able to compensate for differences.
- Socioeconomic Status: Some studies have indicated that there may be more children from lower socioeconomic levels with speech problems than there are from higher socioeconomic levels. However, it is possible that the findings have been confounded by the type of language stimulation and reinforcement received by these children.
- Personality: Within the broad range of normal psychological profiles, personality does not appear to have a causal relationship to speech sound production.

However, there are some indications that children with severe speech sound disorders have more adjustment and behavioral problems than other children do.

In summary, causes generally are not readily found for speech sound errors. Therefore, they do not usually play an important role in therapy (McReynolds, 1986). However, as will be noted in the following section, causes continue to be searched for during an assessment in case a correctable cause does exist.

Assessment

What Happens During an Assessment?

If a child has failed a screening, the next step (with parental permission) is an individual diagnostic session. Such an assessment for speech sound errors might include (1) a case history, (2) an oral peripheral examination, (3) a hearing screening, (4) an articulation test, (5) a phonological assessment, (6) a conversational speech or oral reading sample, (7) a measure of auditory discrimination, and (8) a measure of stimulability. These measures may be assessed by standardized tests or by materials and/or local norms developed by the speech-language pathologist. A speech sample may be tape recorded for later analysis, particularly if abnormal phonological processes are suspected. Phonological analyses can be very time consuming and can be particularly difficult to score if more than one process occurs in the same word. Generally they are only conducted when multiple speech sound errors are present. To save time, some speech-language pathologists will use a computer program to help analyze data.

Does It Really Make a Difference Whether a Problem Is One of Articulation or Phonology?

Yes, because therapeutic goals and procedures are different.

Then How Can Articulatory Disorders Be Differentiated from Phonological Disorders?

The information gathered during an assessment will be analyzed and a decision will be made as to whether a problem, if indeed a problem does exist, is articulatory or phonological in nature. It is not the purpose here to delve into details of such an analysis, but it should prove useful to discuss several general indicators:

1. Children with phonological disorders are more apt to make multiple sound errors (resulting in reduced intelligibility), whereas children with articulatory problems are more likely to err on only a few sounds.

2. The errors exhibited by children with phonological disorders generally fall into a pattern that is explained by the phonological process. Examples:
   a. A child makes an error on a sound in one position but produces it correctly in another position, demonstrating that he or she possesses the motoric ability to produce the sound, yet he does not produce it in all of the proper places. For example, a child may omit "g" in "dog" but produce "g" in "go" (final consonant deletion).
   b. A child makes mistakes on whole classes of sounds, such as substituting stops for all fricatives (stopping).
3. Children with phonological disorders are likely to have other language delays. (Remember that phonology is the sound component of language.)

Will a Child Outgrow a Problem?

There is no sure way of determining this. Nevertheless, an attempt is made to determine whether or not a problem exists for a particular child with regard to that child's chronological age (refer back to the sound acquisition guidelines on page 35). If it is determined that errors are within normal limits, the child may be said to have *maturational* or *developmental* speech sound errors. If results are borderline, the child may be retested at a later date(s) in order to document progress or lack of progress in speech sound acquisition. Sometimes this is called *tracking*.

It is possible that the more problems children have in other developmental areas, such as motor, cognitive, and social areas, the less likely they are to "outgrow" speech sound errors (Shriberg, 1980). Other factors sometimes considered in determining how likely a child is to outgrow a problem include consistency of error, stimulability for the correct production, and type of error. A consistent articulation error (i.e., the erred-on sound is essentially always wrong) is less apt to be affected by maturational processes (outgrown) than is an inconsistent error. The fact that the error is inconsistent may signify that the sound is being acquired.

Auditory and visual clues may be used, along with specific directions, to test stimulability. For example, in order to stimulate a child to produce the "s" sound, the child may be directed to watch and listen carefully as the speech-language pathologist says the sound. The child is then asked to produce the sound. If the sound is still not correct, instructions, such as "place your tongue tip near the ridge behind your front teeth, loosely bite your back teeth together, and blow gently," may be given. A child who is not stimulable (i.e., with help still cannot produce a sound correctly) is less apt to acquire a sound without intervention than a child who is stimulable. However, if the child is stimulable, it is no guarantee that the sound will be acquired without therapy (Schwartz, 1983). On the other hand, stimulability can be an important prognosticator; if a child is stimulable and is enrolled in therapy, success and progress may be relatively rapid.

"Type of error" refers primarily to lateral lisps, distorted slushy productions of "s," "z," "sh," "zh," "ch," and/or "j as in jam." Children who lateralize these sounds are far less apt to correct them on their own than are children who have frontal lisps (the substitution of voiceless and voiced "th" for some or all of these sounds).

Treatment

Articulation

What Is the Goal of Articulation Therapy?

The goal in articulation therapy is for a child to learn to motorically produce correct speech sounds in all speaking situations. In other words, a child must learn how to position and move the articulators to produce a sound. Therapy can be broadly conceptualized as having two subgoals: (1) the acquisition of (or the ability to produce) the correct sound and (2) the habituation of that correct sound in all contexts and speaking situations (*carryover* or *generalization*).

Some speech-language pathologists will add a third subgoal that can be referred to as *maintenance*. This refers to the time period after a child has been dismissed from therapy. In other words, some speech-language pathologists distinguish between the time that a child is habituating a sound(s) while still enrolled in therapy and the time that a child continues to habituate a sound(s) after dismissal from therapy. In the interest of simplification, only the first two subgoals will be addressed in this book.

What Sound Should a Child Work on First?

If a child has more than one error sound, the speech-language pathologist will decide which sound to begin with by considering a number of factors that may include the following:

- The normal progression of speech sound development. This refers to the relationship between speech sound acquisition and age.
- The sounds used most frequently in children's speech. The more frequent an error is, the more noticeable it is.
- A sound that is important for personal reasons. The sounds in a child's name may be given preferential consideration. The parents or teacher may request that a particular sound be worked on in therapy.
- Visible sounds. Sounds that are more visible are easier to learn than sounds that are less visible.
- A sound that a child can produce correctly in at least one word. The speech-language pathologist may be able to use this word to stimulate correct production in other words.
- The sound that will contribute the most to increased intelligibility. This may be closely related to the frequency of occurrence of a sound in a child's speech, although type of error (omission, substitution, or distortion) may also be a factor.
- The sound for which quickest success is anticipated. This will relate to some of the above factors, primarily visibility of sound and ability to produce the sound in at least one word.
- Cognates. Pairs of sounds that differ only by the presence or absence of voicing will be worked on simultaneously. Frequently, as children learn to produce one sound of a pair correctly, they naturally become able to produce the other.

- Nonemergent, nonstimulable sounds that are phonetically more complex may produce the most change in the child's speech, i.e., on both sounds specifically taught as well as sounds not taught (Gierut, Morrisette, Hughes, & Rowland, 1996; Powell, Elbert, & Dinnsen, 1991; Tyler & Figurski, 1994).

Just What Goes on in Therapy?

Traditional articulation therapy involves discrimination and production. *Discrimination* is the ability to differentiate (1) between different sounds and (2) between correct productions and distorted productions of sounds. Depending on the philosophy and training of the speech-language pathologist and the needs of the child, differing degrees of emphasis and time in therapy may be placed on discrimination tasks. *Production* refers to the ability to produce a sound either alone or in various contexts.

Therapy involves a gradual progression from less to more difficult and lengthy contexts and can be divided into various stages including:

1. Isolation (all alone, with no other sound)
2. Syllables
3. Words (first one-syllable words containing only one target sound, i.e., the sound to be corrected, then multisyllabic words and words containing more than one target sound; e.g., for the "s" sound, "soap" would be followed by "lesson" and "seesaw")
4. Phrases or short sentences containing only one word with the target sound (e.g., for the "s" sound, "I want some")
5. Longer sentences containing more than one word with the target sound (e.g., for the "s" sound, "Did you see the six new posters in Mrs. Brown's office?")
6. Reading
7. Structured conversation (the child is provided a topic to discuss)
8. Unstructured spontaneous conversation

Following this sequence, a child would first learn to produce a sound all alone with no other sound, then progress to production of the sound in syllables, and so forth.

Teachers may hear a speech-language pathologist refer to the ability of a child to produce sounds in the initial (prevocalic), medial (intervocalic), or final (postvocalic) position (e.g., "ch" is in the initial position of "choose," the medial position of "teacher," and the final position of "which"). Most speech-language pathologists feel that, with the possible exception of "r" and "er," production is easiest in the initial position and hardest in the medial position. Thus, after production in isolation, they have a child attempt to produce a sound in syllables, first in the initial position, then in the final position, and last in the medial position. Some speech-language pathologists begin work on the production of "r" in the initial position and the syllabic consonant "er" in the final position.

There are a number of specific therapeutic approaches to articulation therapy. Most speech-language pathologists work eclectically, pulling from various therapeutic approaches the techniques they feel are best for a particular child at a particular time.

Are Some Sounds Harder to Learn Than Others?

It certainly takes longer to teach some sounds than others. Part of the reason may lie in the amount of visual, tactile (sense of touch), and kinesthetic (sense of movement and posture) feedback that is present for a given sound. This may sound complicated, but consider the "voiceless th" and "r" sounds.

Frequently the production of the "voiceless th" sound in isolation can be taught in just a few minutes with a mirror and the directions: "Watch me and listen to the way I say this sound." (Then say "voiceless th.") "Now look in the mirror and you try it. Stick the tip of your tongue out between your teeth and blow gently."

On the other hand, say "er" and think about the instructions that could be given to a child who cannot say the sound. The sound is not really visible, so watching the instructor or looking in the mirror will not help much. Say "er" and think about where your tongue is. Compared to the "voiceless th," placement is much more difficult to describe. Most of the tongue, including the tip, is not even touching another part of the mouth. To further confuse the issue, there are two possible tongue positions that will result in a correctly produced "er" sound and, generally, one of these is much easier for a child to use than the other. However, there is no way to know for sure which set of directions to start with for any one child.

Phonology

What Is the Goal When a Problem Is One of Phonology?

Because many of a child's errors fall into one process, the goal of remediation is to eliminate that process. For example, the goal may be to eliminate the final consonant deletion process. Rather than the goal being to correct just one sound or a cognate pair of sounds, as it is in articulation therapy, the goal is for a child to use a more adult form of communication (i.e., without the phonological process) for increased intelligibility.

Just What Goes on in Therapy?

To continue with the final consonant deletion example, assume that a child deletes eight different sounds when they occur in the final position of words. Even though the goal is to eliminate the process of final consonant deletion, in therapy the child will not work on all eight sounds but a subgroup of these eight. The assumption is that the child will learn (1) that there is a rule that says that final consonants should not be omitted or, in effect, that final consonants are important, and (2) that this rule will generalize to the other consonants not directly included in the therapy lessons. This is presumed to be more efficient than working on each of the eight sounds separately.

One approach to this problem would be to use what is called *minimally contrastive words* or *minimal contrasts*. (A pair of such words might be called *minimal pairs*.) A list of such words could include "sea, seed, seal, seam, seat." Therapy is set up so that in order to respond correctly, children must use the information contained in the final consonant. For example, children are rewarded when (1) they follow directions (e.g., when confronted with a group of pictures, they respond correctly to an instruction, such as "put the (*seal*) in your pile of cards") or (2) they speak plainly enough that the speech-language pathologist follows their directions (e.g., a child instructs the speech-language pathologist to "give me the (*seed*)"). Notice that work did not begin with the sound in isolation, as it usually does in articulation therapy, but began in a meaningful linguistic context. In this way, children use information about a correct sound in a language context and learn that there are consequences related to their language behavior. (Remember that phonology is one component of language.)

Work on stopping might involve contrasting short (as are stop sounds) versus long (as are fricative sounds) nonspeech activities, such as drawing short lines versus long lines and then adding sound while drawing these lines. Frequently children who originally substituted "t" for "s" in words such as "soup," "soap," "sun," and "sandwich" will not necessarily learn to make the correct "s" sound but will begin to use the typical "voiceless th" substitution for the "s," which does eliminate the phonological process of stopping and, most importantly, increases intelligibility. For many children the "th" for "s" substitution will be age appropriate and is acceptable for the time being.

Work on discrimination as well as production may be necessary. Furthermore, therapeutic procedures for articulatory and phonological disorders are not necessarily incompatible. Both may be used simultaneously with a particular child. For example, some children may need instructions about how to produce a sound to be able to produce it correctly in a particular context (even though they produce it correctly in other contexts).

A child may demonstrate more than one phonological process in speech. If so, the speech-language pathologist will need to determine which ones, if any, might normally still be present for a particular child.

In determining this, the speech-language pathologist should consider, as recommended by ASHA (Cole, 1983), not only guidelines or norms established from published research, which tends to use predominately white children as subjects, but also local norms that the speech-language pathologist has established. For example, Haynes and Moran (1989) found that rural black children in Alabama who spoke the African American dialect of that region continued to use final consonant deletion in a normal manner beyond the time that would be expected for children speaking Standard American English.

If there is more than one phonological process that should no longer be present, then a decision about which process(es) to target first in therapy will need to be made. Several factors will be considered, including how frequently the process occurs in the child's speech, which one interferes most with intelligibility, which one should have been deleted first (i.e., the one that reflects the most immaturity), which one would the child have the quickest success eliminating, and which one would produce the most change in the child's communicative abilities. Sometimes therapy is planned so that two processes are targeted at the same time; half of the therapy session is spent working on one process and half on the other. Another approach is cyclic; that is, one process is targeted for a certain number of hours, sessions, or weeks, then a different process, perhaps yet a different process, and then back to the first process.

When Should Children Be Dismissed from Therapy?

Many states and school districts have dismissal criteria that IEP committees can use in making a termination decision. Children whose disability no longer exists or who cannot be expected to continue to make progress because of physical or physiological limitations should obviously be dismissed. For some children it is a judgment call. An IEP committee could wait until children made absolutely no errors before dismissing them from therapy. However, research has indicated that a child need not be performing at the 100 percent criterion in order to be dismissed. When children are dismissed while still making some errors, they generally continue to improve. This is certainly more time and cost efficient. However, whether a particular child should be dismissed when able to produce a sound correctly 80 percent, 90 percent, or 95 percent of the time, or some other percentage, has not been conclusively determined.

Toward the end of therapy, a speech-language pathologist may recommend to the IEP committee that the number of sessions be decreased or that the monitoring service delivery option be used to help prevent regressing or backsliding. Monitoring can be accomplished by talking to the child for a few minutes, by checking with the teacher or parents, or by unobtrusively listening to the child.

How Can a Teacher Help Children with Articulatory or Phonological Problems?

A teacher can be supportive of a child's efforts in therapy by:

1. Encouraging the child to go to therapy and to be on time.
2. Showing an interest in what the child is doing in therapy. This is especially easy if a child has a speech therapy notebook that can be shared with the teacher.
3. Not demanding (or even asking) that a child say a word correctly before the speech-language pathologist has told the teacher that the child is ready to produce the necessary sound(s) correctly. In other words, it takes time before success in therapy is translated into better speech in the classroom, and a teacher does not want to demand better speech before a child is capable of it.
4. Recognizing that even after a child is capable of producing a sound in some contexts, the child may still be unable to produce it in other contexts. For example, just because a child can say a good "s" in the word "so" or even in the longer word "summer" does not mean that the child can say the "s" sounds in "mistakes," "Mississippi," or "scarce." Do not accuse a child of not trying

unless you know from the speech-language pathologist that the child is capable of the task.

5. Helping a child remember to use correct sounds during carryover. The teacher and speech-language pathologist should consult to determine exactly how this help should be rendered for each child. Possibilities include just listening and praising a child for good speech, or an occasional unobtrusive signal when the teacher hears a child misarticulating. Under no circumstances, however, should the teacher attempt to correct a child every time an error is made. For one thing, the teacher does not have the time to do this and, more importantly, the child may easily become embarrassed, frustrated, and self-conscious. This could result in the child talking less, which is certainly not a goal.

6. Being aware of increased numbers of errors (backsliding) after a child has been dismissed from therapy and contacting the speech-language pathologist, who can follow up on the problem.

7. Accepting young children's maturational or developmental speech sound errors. If prognostic tests indicate that the odds are with a child "growing out" of a problem, therapy would be superfluous.

8. Discouraging other children from teasing a child about either the errors or the fact that the child receives therapy.

9. Setting a good example. Speak well yourself.

10. Modeling good articulation by allowing the child to hear at least part of his or her message correctly said. This is especially important in the earlier grades.

Is There a Relationship Between Speech Sound Errors and Academic Subjects?

Yes. Research has not yet clearly explained the relationship, but a relationship is there. Several studies have shown that children with articulation disorders are at risk for academic problems, especially in reading, spelling, and written language, even after they have corrected their articulation errors. Similarly, studies have shown that young children with phonological disorders are more apt to have problems in other areas of language and academic problems (Blachman, 1989; Bradley, 1988; Kamhi & Catts, 1989; Hoffman, 1990, 1992; Lewis, O'Donnell, Freebairn, & Taylor, 1998; Lundberg, 1988; Stewart, Gonzales, & Page, 1997).

A major part of the relationship may lie in the association between awareness skills and production (Harbers, Paden, & Halle, 1999). Phonological awareness refers to the ability to think about and manipulate phonological segments. More simply put, it involves knowledge about words, syllables, and phonemes and the ability to manipulate syllables and phonemes. Good phonological awareness skills are positively correlated with academic success, and training in phonological awareness to improve these skills can result in improved reading abilities (Stewart, Gonzales, & Page, 1997). Swank and Catts (1994) even found that phonological awareness skills correlated higher with reading ability than did measures of verbal and nonverbal intelligence.

So what are some of the phonological awareness skills that can have such an effect on reading, spelling, and written language? Examples include (Merritt & Culatta, 1998):

- Identifying words or the number of words said or written
- Identifying which words are longer and which are shorter
- Counting syllables
- Deleting syllables
- Rhyming activities, such as picking out from a group of words the one word that does not rhyme with the others
- Discriminating between phonemes (speech sounds)
- Discriminating between initial consonants (called the onset) and the rest of the word (called the rime)
- Working with word families ("bat, mat, cat, fat, rat, sat") in which children identify similarities and differences
- Identifying individual phonemes (this is generally easiest after exposure to print)
- Identifying sound families, such as sibilants or stops (names, such as hissy or windy sounds for sibilants and pop-pop-pop sounds for the stops can be used to make this easier)
- Counting phonemes
- Deleting phonemes
- Blending phonemes

Phonological awareness progresses from larger units to smaller units, that is, from sentences to words to syllables to sounds. Thus, Merritt and Culatta (1998) advise that not only should teachers begin with the larger units, but that they should also begin with sounds that are learned first in normal sound acquisition, begin with easier tasks and move toward harder tasks, teach manner and place of production, and work with a small group of sounds at a time. Phonological awareness skills can and should be taught at the preschool level on until children become literate. Thus, whole-class activities would be appropriate at the preschool, kindergarten, and first grade levels. Then, when certain children have been identified as having reading difficulties, they could be given extra help in small groups with the phonological awareness skills that they have difficulty with but that their classmates have mastered. In Gillon and Dodd's study (1995), even 10- and 12-year-old children with reading difficulties improved their reading accuracy and comprehension through explicit instruction in phonological awareness.

More and more resources are becoming available to help assess and teach phonological awareness. Informally, invented spelling gives an indication of children's phonological awareness. Merritt and Culatta (1998) provide a list of formal assessment instruments that can be used to identify children's needs and document progress, as well as examples of activities for teaching phonological awareness. van Kleeck, Gillam, and McFadden (1998) also provide examples of sequential phoneme awareness activities involving initial sounds, final sounds, and blends for preschoolers and early elementary students. Teachers and speech-language pathologists should share their knowledge and work together to help children with poor phonological awareness skills.

What about the Articulation and Phonology of Students Who Speak Dialects or English as a Second Language?

In the United States, *Standard American English (SAE)* is the language of power and money. It is used by the media, the government, and most businesses. Many of our children have had little or no exposure to SAE when they enter school. Instead, they enter our schools speaking a dialect or another language. A *dialect* is any form of a base language that has a rule-governed structure. It is spoken by a distinct sub-population of those who use the base language. This subpopulation may be identified with a particular geographical region, socioeconomic level, ethnicity, or culture.

When children speak a foreign language as the first or native language, we say they speak English as a second language (ESL). For many of these children the first language will be the home language and English the school language. If children speak some English but not well, the term *limited English proficiency (LEP)* is used. According to the U.S. Bureau of the Census, 14 percent of school-age children speak English as a second language; their first language is most often Spanish or one of the Asian languages.

There is some disagreement about whether *African American English (AAE)*, previously called Black English (BE) and Black English Vernacular (BEV) and also currently referred to as *ebonics* (from *ebony* plus *phonics*), is a language of its own or a dialect of SAE. Robert Williams (Love, 1997), a black psychologist who coined the term *ebonics*, has described it as a combination of English vocabulary and African language structure. He noted that American black speakers tended to drop certain consonants from blends, especially at the ends of words, and that the typical phonetic pattern was consonant, vowel, consonant, vowel, and so on.

All educators are challenged by the significant increase in minority populations that do not speak Standard American English as a first language, because for the most part this is what we teach. Moreover, this increase is predicted to continue. The issue is compounded by a shortage of teachers and speech-language pathologists who are proficient in any language besides SAE.

Many believe that the first language or dialect should be preserved, because it serves a social purpose in the community of speakers speaking that language or dialect, allowing the child to communicate effectively with that community and to belong to that community (Campbell, 1993). This view celebrates diversity yet recognizes that at times the child (and later the adult) may need or want to be able to use SAE to effectively communicate in other settings. If the speech-language pathologist is not proficient in the child's language or dialect, someone (such as someone else in the school system, a parent, or a community member) must be found who can provide information about that language or dialect.

The following examples will highlight some (but not all) of the common articulatory and phonological differences between SAE and AAE and between SAE and Spanish, the second most frequently spoken language in the United States, which has several dialects each based on the country of origin.

African American English can be characterized by:

- "d" substituted for "voiced th" at the beginnings of words, such as "dem" for "them," and "d" or "v" substituted for "voiced th" in the middle or at the ends of words, such as "mudder" for "mother"
- "t" or "f" substituted for "voiceless th" especially in the middle and at the ends of words, such as "toof" for "tooth"
- "l" deleted in some contexts, such as hep for help
- Unstressed initial syllables deleted, such as "member" for "remember"
- "r" weaker or deleted depending on the context, such as "cah" for "car"
- "b" substituted for "v," such as "bery" for "very"
- Final consonants weakened
- "skr" substituted for "str," such as "skreet" for "street"
- "gonna" substituted for "going to"
- One consonant of a consonant blend omitted at the end of a word, such as "bes" for "best"
- Nasal consonant omitted at the end of a word, such as "ma" for "man"

Spanish is characterized by:

- Five vowels and four diphthongs compared to 12 vowels and five diphthongs in English, so errors on English vowels may occur
- An absence of final consonant clusters, such as "st" in "last" and "lk" in "milk," so the final consonant cluster in English may be omitted or distorted
- Only 18 consonants, which include two not used in English (native Spanish speakers are most apt to make substitution or distortion errors on "ng," "j as in jam,", "ch," "y as in yo-yo," "voiced th," "voiceless th," and "v")
- A different *prosody* (the melody of speech perceived as stress and intonation), in which all vowels have the same length instead of vowel length being determined by syllable stress

Case Histories

Jill

Jill, a third-grader, had been enrolled in speech therapy for approximately 4 months. She had problems with the articulation of the "r," "s," and "z" sounds. The word "ride," for example, was spoken as "wide," "soup" as "thoup," and "zoo" as "thoo." Sounds were misarticulated consistently and in all positions. Jill was a bright girl and did excellent work in the classroom. She was well adjusted and accepted by her peers.

Jill was cooperative in speech therapy sessions, but there seemed to be almost no progress toward correcting the misarticulated sounds. Not until a second conference was held with the parents and teacher to review the IEP was it learned that correct articulation was being negatively reinforced. Specifically, it was learned that Jill's father and an older sibling had been imitating Jill's faulty articulation since she began to talk. For some reason they thought this was of no harm and rather "cute," as the mother expressed it.

Several weeks after the imitation of Jill's misarticulation ceased, Jill started to make good progress toward correcting her faulty sounds. At the end of the school year, Jill actually had attained almost 100 percent mastery of the "r," "s," and "z" sounds in spontaneous speech.

Michael

Michael was first seen as a 4-year, 8-month-old preschooler because his mother said that he was hard to understand. This was an understatement. Here is a summary of his articulation test results:

List # 1:   He could say the consonant sounds "p," "b," "m," "n," "w," "t," "d," "y as in yo-yo," and "ng."

List # 2:   He was unable to say the consonant sounds "h," "k," "f," "g," "sh," "ch," "j as in jam," "l," "r," "voiced th," "voiceless th," "v," "zh," "s," and "z."

For words that began with sounds from the #2 list, Michael substituted sounds that he could produce from list #1, except for the sound "h," which he always omitted. The "t" was a favorite sound, and he used it for "k," "j as in jam," "ch," "sh," and "voiceless th." He used "d" for "g" and "voiced th"; "p" for "f"; and "b" for "v." Thus, some of his words were: <u>tee</u> for key, see, tree; <u>tam</u> for jam; <u>too</u> for chew, shoe, school, glue; <u>toe</u> for show, slow; <u>tum</u> for thumb; <u>doe</u> for go, goat; <u>dem</u> for them; <u>punny</u> for funny; <u>ow</u> for house; <u>oh</u> for hose; <u>uh</u> for hug; <u>pea</u> for please, piece; and <u>we</u> for leaf. When List #2 sounds occurred in the middle of words or at the ends of words, he generally just omitted them. He used one consonant for two- and three-consonant blends. Often the one consonant present was not one that was a part of the blend but a consonant that was being substituted for one of the actual consonants. For example, he said "pie" for "fly" because he substituted "p" for "f" and omitted the "l." Furthermore, he had many language errors. For example, he always substituted *me*, *him*, *her*, and *them* for *I*, *he*, *she*, and *they* and omitted most linking and helping verbs and the articles *the*, *an*, and *a*.

Therapy was both articulation-based and phonology-based. One of his articulation goals was to learn how to make some of the sounds that he could not say, such as "k" and "g." One of the phonology goals was to learn to produce consonants that could be prolonged (the phonology process to be eliminated was stridency deletion). It has been 2 years since therapy began, and Michael is now in the first grade. Sometimes the listener can easily understand him but at other times must pay attention and think in order to understand him. He now uses "k," "g," "f," "h," and "l" consistently and uses the "voiceless th" inconsistently for the "s," "sh," and "ch" sounds and the "voiced th" for the "z" and "j as in jam" sounds, which are age-appropriate substitutions. He continues to use one consonant for two- and three-consonant blends. Language-wise, he generally uses the nominative pronouns correctly but still omits linking and helping verbs about 30 percent of the time. Academically he is having difficulty in the language/reading areas. He cannot name most of the letters of the alphabet and has little consistent knowledge of what letters make what sounds. Mathematics is much easier. His IQ is in the normal to low normal range.

Summary

Some Important Points to Remember

- A speech sound is called a phoneme and is the smallest segment of a word.
- IPA is the International Phonetic Alphabet and represents sounds.
- A diphthong is made when the articulators move from one vowel to another within the same syllable.
- There are approximately 17 vowel sounds.
- Some consonants are produced with voice and others without voice, as in "b" and "p."
- Children make several types of speech sound errors: distortions, substitutions, omissions, and additions.
- Speech sound errors can affect the intelligibility of the message.
- Some speech sound errors are consistent and some are inconsistent.
- There are articulatory errors and phonological errors.
- There is a natural developmental sequence in speech sound development.
- Phonology involves the study of speech sounds and the rules for combining them.
- The most commonly misarticulated sounds are "s," "z," and "r."
- Phonological awareness skills can help a child develop literacy.
- Assessment of a speech sound problem might involve a case history, an oral peripheral examination, a hearing screening, an articulation test, a stimulability test, and a conversational speech or reading sample.
- Phonological disorders are likely to be characterized by multiple sound production problems.
- There is no sure way of determining the extent to which a child will outgrow a sound production problem.
- Inconsistent errors are more likely to be outgrown than consistent ones.
- Stimulability is a good prognosticator of whether or not a child will outgrow a sound production problem.

- The more developmental problems a child has, the less likely he or she is to outgrow a speech problem.
- Consideration of several factors determine which sound or phonological process is worked on first in therapy.
- Articulation therapy progresses from shorter units, such as sounds, to longer units, such as sentences.
- The more severe the articulatory or phonological problem, the more likely the child will have difficulty with other language-based tasks, such as reading and writing.
- Some sounds are more difficult to learn than others; "r," for example, is more difficult than the "voiceless th."
- The aim of phonology therapy is to work on a sound process rather than to correct a particular sound.
- The goals of articulation therapy are to produce correct sounds and to stabilize use of correct sounds in all speech.
- Phonological therapy utilizes linguistic contexts.

"Do"s and "Don't"s for Teachers

"Do"s

- Refer a child who is difficult to understand to a speech-language pathologist, regardless of the child's age.
- Work closely with the speech-language pathologist when working with a child with a speech sound problem.
- Attempt to reinforce in the classroom what a child has mastered in the therapy sessions.
- Cooperate fully with a speech-language pathologist when he or she wishes to recheck a child who has been in therapy.
- Encourage the child.

"Don't"s

- Don't permit ridicule of a child with a speech sound problem.
- Don't demand correction of age-appropriate maturational errors or errors that the speech-language pathologist has not yet indicated have been mastered.

Self-Test

True or False

1. In this chapter, IPA stands for the Independent Phonetic Alphabet.   _____

2. A phoneme is a speech sound.   _____

3. A diphthong is a sound that results from articulatory movement from one   _____
   vowel to another vowel within the same syllable.

4. When a child says "wed" for "red," the type of error made is one of substitution.   _____

5. Intelligibility of speech is not affected by disorders of articulation.   _____

6. As many as one-fourth of all first-graders may misarticulate one or more speech sounds.   _____

7. *Maturational* or *developmental articulatory errors* is a term that refers to speech sound errors that may be "outgrown."   _____

8. Phonology is a component of language.   _____

9. Phonological development is not rule-based.   _____

10. Auditory discrimination has little or nothing to do with either articulatory or phonological problems.   _____

11. Phonological disorders can be distinguished from articulatory disorders.   _____

12. An error of articulation that is consistent in the speech of a child is less likely to be outgrown than an inconsistent error.   _____

13. "Sea, seed, seal, seam, seat" are examples of minimally contrastive words.   _____

14. A child should not be dismissed from therapy until 100 percent of the phonological or articulatory problems are corrected.   _____

References

Bernthal, J. E., & Bankson, N. W. (1981). *Articulation Disorders*. Englewood Cliffs, NJ: Prentice-Hall.

Blachman, B. (1989). Phonological awareness and word recognition. In A. Kamhi & H. Catts (Eds.), *Reading disabilities: A developmental language perspective*. Boston: College-Hill.

Bradley, L. (1988). Rhyme recognition and reading and spelling in young children. In R. Masland & M. Masland (Eds.), *Preschool prevention of reading failure*. Parkton, MD: York Press.

Campbell, L. (1993). Maintaining the integrity of home linguistic varieties: Black English vernacular. *American Journal of Speech-Language Pathology, 2*, 11–12.

Churchill, J. D., Hodson, B. W., Jones, B. W., & Novak, R. E. (1988). Phonological systems of speech-disordered clients with positive/negative histories of otitis media. *Language, Speech, and Hearing Services in Schools, 19*, 100–107.

Cole, L. (1983). Implications of the position on social dialects. *ASHA, 25*(9), 25–27.

Crowe-Hall, B. J. (1991). Attitudes of fourth and sixth graders toward peers with mild articulation disorders. *Language, Speech, and Hearing Services in Schools, 22*, 334–340.

Edwards, M. L., & Shriberg, L. D. (1983). *Phonology: Applications in communicative disorders*. San Diego, CA: College-Hill.

Gierut, J. A., Morrisette, M. L., Hughes, M. T., & Rowland, S. (1996). Phonological treatment efficacy and developmental norms. *Language, Speech, and Hearing Services in Schools, 27*, 215–230.

Gillon, G., & Dodd, B. (1995). The effects of training phonological, semantic, and syntactic processing skills in spoken language on reading ability. *Language, Speech, and Hearing Services in Schools, 26*, 58–68.

Haelsig, P. C., & Madison, C. L. (1986). A study of phonological processes exhibited by 3-, 4-, and 5-year old children. *Language, Speech, and Hearing Services in Schools, 17*, 107–114.

Harbers, H. M., Paden, E. P., & Halle, J. W. (1999). Phonological awareness and production: Changes during intervention. *Language, Speech, and Hearing Services in Schools, 30,* 50–60.

Haynes, W. O., & Moran, M. (1989). A cross-sectional developmental study of final consonant production in southern black children from preschool through third grade. *Language, Speech, and Hearing Services in Schools, 20,* 400–406.

Hodson, B. W. (1980). *The assessment of phonological processes.* Danville, IL: Interstate.

Hodson, B. W. (1992). Applied phonology: Constructs, contributions, and issues. *Language, Speech, and Hearing Services in Schools, 23,* 247–253.

Hoffman, P. (1990). Spelling, phonology, and the speech-language pathologist: A whole language perspective. *Language, Speech, and Hearing Services in Schools, 21,* 238–243.

Hoffman, P. R. (1992). Synergistic development of phonetic skill. *Language, Speech, and Hearing Services in Schools, 23,* 254–260.

Ingram, D. (1976). *Phonological disability in children.* London: Arnold.

Kamhi, A., & Catts, H. (1989). *Reading disabilities: A developmental language perspective.* Boston: College-Hill.

Lewis, B. A., O'Donnell, B., Freebairn, L. A., & Taylor, H. G. (1998). Spoken language and written expression—Interplay of delays. *American Journal of Speech-Language Pathology, 7,* 77–84.

Love, A. A. (1997). *Consonant, vowel. That's African.* Lafayette, IN: Journal and Courier.

Lundberg, I. (1988). Preschool prevention of reading failure: Does training in phonological awareness work? In R. Masland & M. Masland (Eds.), *Preschool prevention of reading failure.* Parkton, MD: York Press.

McReynolds, L. V. (1986). Functional articulation disorders. In G. H. Shames & E. H. Wiig (Eds.), *Human communication disorders* (2nd ed.) (pp. 139–182). Columbus, OH: Merrill.

Merritt, D. D., & Culatta, B. (1998). *Language intervention in the classroom.* San Diego, CA: Singular.

Mowrer, D. E., Wahl, P., & Doolan, S. J. (1978). Effect of lisping on audience evaluation of male speakers. *Journal of Speech and Hearing Disorders, 43,* 140–148.

Pendergast, K. (1966). Articulation study of 15,255 Seattle first-grade children with and without kindergarten. *Exceptional Child, 32,* 541–547.

Perrin, E. H. (1954). The social position of the speech defective child. *Journal of Speech and Hearing Disorders, 19,* 250–252.

Powell, T. W., Elbert, M., & Dinnsen, D. A. (1991). Stimulability as a factor in the phonologic generalization of misarticulating preschool children. *Journal of Speech and Hearing Research, 34,* 1318–1328.

Schwartz, R. G. (1983). Diagnosis of speech sound disorders in children. In I. J. Meitus & B. Weinberg (eds.), *Diagnosis in speech-language pathology* (pp. 113–149). Baltimore, MD: University Park Press.

Shriberg, L. D. (1980). Developmental phonological disorders. In T. J. Hixon, L. D. Shriberg, & J. H. Saxman (Eds.), *Introduction to communication disorders* (pp. 263–309). Englewood Cliffs, NJ: Prentice-Hall.

Silverman, E. (1976). Listeners' impressions of speakers with lateral lisps. *Journal of Speech and Hearing Disorders, 41,* 547–552.

Silverman, F. (1986). Documenting the impact of a mild dysarthria on peer perception (Letter to the editor). *Language, Speech, and Hearing Services in School, 17,* 143.

Silverman, F. H., & Falk, S. M. (1992). Attitudes of teenagers toward peers who have a single articulation error. *Language, Speech, and Hearing Services in Schools, 23,* 187–188.

Silverman, F. H., & Paulus, P. G. (1989). Peer reactions to teenagers who substitute /w/ for /r/. *Language, Speech, and Hearing Services in Schools, 20,* 219–221.

Stewart, S. R., Gonzalez, L. S., & Page, J. L. (1997). Incidental learning of sight words during articulation training. *Language, Speech, and Hearing Services in Schools, 28,* 115–126.

Stoel-Gammon, C., & Dunn, C. (1985). *Normal and disordered phonology in children.* Baltimore, MD: University Park Press.

Swank, L. K., & Catts, H. W. (1994). Phonological awareness and written word decoding. *Language, Speech, and Hearing Services in Schools, 25,* 9–14.

Tyler, A. A., & Figurski, G. R. (1994). Phonetic inventory changes after treating distinctions along an implicational hierarchy. *Clinical Linguistics and Phonetics, 8,* 91–107.

van Kleeck, A., Gillam, R. B., & McFadden, T. U. (1998). A study of classroom based phonological awareness training for preschoolers with speech and/or language disorders. *American Journal of Speech-Language Pathology, 7,* 65–76.

Webster, P. E., & Plante, A. S. (1992). Effects of phonological impairment on word, syllable, and phoneme segmentation and reading. *Language, Speech, and Hearing Services in Schools, 23,* 176–182.

Chapter 3

<hr/>

Language Disabilities

Language is a rule-based code that we learn and use in order to communicate our ideas and express our wants and needs. The definition of language proposed by the American Speech-Language-Hearing Association (ASHA) helps identify the components of language. The definition states

> Language is a complex and dynamic system of conventional symbols that is used in various modes for thought and communication. Contemporary views of human language hold that:
>
> - language evolves within specific historical, social, and cultural contexts
> - language, as rule governed behavior, is described by at least five parameters— phonologic, morphologic, syntactic, semantic, and pragmatic
> - language learning and use are determined by the interaction of biological, cognitive, psychosocial, and environmental factors
> - effective use of language for communication requires a broad understanding of human interaction including such associated factors as nonverbal cues, motivation, and sociocultural roles (ASHA Committee on Language, 1983, p. 44)

You should particularly note the five parameters. The phonologic parameter (speech sounds and speech sound sequences) was discussed in Chapter 2. The other four will be explored in this chapter. Although the terms *form, content*, and *use* coined by Bloom and Lahey (1978) will not be emphasized in this book, readers should be familiar with them because they are often referred to. Form includes phonology, morphology, and syntax. Content includes semantics, and use refers to pragmatics.

Other terms that you may see relating to language are *communicative competence* and *metalinguistic ability*. Communicative competence refers to one's knowledge of all the dimensions of language. It cannot be assessed directly; instead, inferences are made by observing a child's ability to use language receptively and expressively.

Metalinguistic ability refers to one's ability to think about language. It enables one to decide whether a message is acceptable or successful in its intent.

How Do Children Learn Language?

Children learn the language of their environment by listening to those around them and practicing what they hear. By their first birthday, they can speak one to two words clearly enough and consistently enough that parents or caregivers recognize their meanings. They can also follow simple requests, such as "Come here" or "Get your blanket," and respond to simple questions, such as "Where is the ball?" Then, by their second birthday, children are putting three to four words together to form simple sentences and following two requests, such as "Get your doll and put it in the wagon." Language growth continues through the preschool years until by kindergarten age, children should be able to tell a story in a logical sequence and, if exposed, have some counting and alphabet knowledge. Until this point, language has consisted primarily of listening and speaking. Once children enter school, their language experience expands to include reading and writing.

How is this language learning possible? Several theories, models, and hypotheses have been posited. Basically, they boil down to nature versus nurture. The nature end of the continuum assumes that language learning is innate and based on genetics and biological factors, while the nurture end argues that language learning is due to environmental factors. The general consensus today is that the truth lies somewhere in between. Certain biological factors must be present, but children's experiences will help shape their language learning (McLaughlin, 1998).

Just What Is the Relationship Between a Learning Disability and a Language Disability?

Various terms have been used as labels for children having difficulty with language, including *language impairment, language difference, language delay, language disorder, learning disability (LD), language-learning disability* or *language-based learning disability, language deviance, language disability, language-reading disorders,* and *specific language impairment.* Most authors make distinctions among at least some of these terms. Teachers will need to become familiar with the terms and definitions that are used in their own school districts. In this chapter the terms *language disabilities* and *specific language impairment* will be used. Whatever the problem is called, it falls under either *communication disorder* or the broader term *learning disabled (LD),* which are classifications for special education purposes and the allocation of federal funding for schools.

The term *learning disability (LD)* encompasses a wide range of disorders that are manifested through difficulties in the acquisition and use of listening, speaking, reading, writing, reasoning, and mathematical abilities. Previously the terms *minimal brain damage* and *minimal brain dysfunction* were used to refer to what we now call learning disability. Certain children are excluded from having a learning disability. For obvious reasons, children who are hearing impaired, visually impaired, mentally handicapped, emotionally handicapped, or who are reared in a linguistically deprived environment cannot be expected to develop language skills in a normal manner. Even though there is a high probability these children will have problems with language, the term *learning disability* is not used to categorize these children when developing IEPs. A learning disability is presumed to be due to central nervous system dysfunction and is not the direct result of these other conditions. More boys than girls are affected, and the problem is lifelong. Many have average or above average intelligence scores. The National Joint Committee on Learning Disabilities stresses the heterogeneity of the population with learning disabilities. This cannot be overemphasized. Although some problems are common among many children and youth with learning disabilities, each person will display a unique pattern of difficulty with various skills affected in varying degrees of severity.

Relatively few children are identified as learning disabled in the preschool years. Most learning disabilities become apparent when the child starts trying to read, write, and do mathematics. However, a number of children are not identified until the late elementary or junior and senior high years, when language demands become more complex (Peters-Johnson, 1992).

What Causes Language Disabilities?

The factors mentioned as exclusions from the definition of learning disabilities, such as mental handicap and hearing impairment, can cause language problems. Language disorders associated with these factors are said to be secondary to the other condition present. Occasionally children are environmentally deprived and not exposed enough to language to learn it or, at the other extreme, are not given a chance to practice it because people in the environment talk for the child or anticipate the child's needs to such an extent that the child has no need to talk.

But what causes the particular language problems that (1) if diagnosed in the preschool years are first labeled communication disorder and then later on in school (if a problem continues) either remain labeled as a communication disorder or become subsumed under the broader category of learning disability depending on whether or not the child's evaluation scores qualify for the learning disability label or (2) if diagnosed after entering school are either labeled communication disorder when the child's evaluation scores do not qualify for the learning disability category or labeled learning disability (in language) if they do qualify?

The cause of most cases is *developmental*; that is, the disabilities show up as the child grows and develops and are not due to any known cause. They may show up as early as 12 to 15 months when the child should begin talking, or not until the language requirements of the school become more intense along about fourth or fifth grade or even later. The language disability of children who are diagnosed prior to entering kindergarten has been referred to as a speech-language delay, speech-language disorder, speech-language impairment, childhood aphasia, language learning disability, specific language disability, specific expressive language impairment, and specific language impairment (SLI). Schuele and Hadley (1999) suggest that SLI should be the term of choice, and state that it is assumed that the cause involves the psychological mechanism for learning language. Children with SLI present with varying degrees of overall severity and varying degrees of problems within each of the five dimensions of language. Approximately 60 percent of children with SLI will also have articulation/phonology disabilities (Schuele & Hadley, 1999). In Schuele and Hadley's (1999) review of the literature, they concluded that many of these children who continue to have language problems will be reclassified as learning disabled and will have problems through adulthood. The remaining language disabilities are called *acquired* language disorders and may be due to head injuries, strokes, infections, tumors, epilepsy, and other neurological problems.

What Are the Dimensions of Language?

The five dimensions of language are phonology, semantics, morphology, syntax, and pragmatics. Phonology was discussed extensively in Chapter 2; the others will be discussed here.

What Is Semantics?

Semantics deals with the meanings of words (including multiple meanings) and word combinations. The words that we know make up our vocabularies (or lexicons). Words can be thought of as a special code that provides us with a way of labeling things, ideas, and concepts. Each language has its own specific words (labels) that are associated with each possible thing, idea, or concept. We cannot adequately communicate without the labels of common meaning that words provide.

Beginning first-graders should have a vocabulary of approximately 2,500 words (Newhoff & Leonard, 1983; Wiig & Semel, 1984). As they progress through elementary school, their ability to differentiate fine meanings between words (e.g., *love, affection, fondness,* and *adoration*); to comprehend and classify words based on spatial, temporal, familial, disjunctive, and logical relationships (Owens, 1984); and to comprehend abstract words that cannot be perceived by the senses, such as *pride, honor,* and *grief,* increases. Children begin to learn modals (*can, could, may, might, will, would, shall,* and *should*) around age 1 and continue to refine their learning of these words until at least 8 years of age (Bliss, 1987). Word definitions that are context bound (i.e., tied to a particular sentence) become more abstract (more like a dictionary definition that is not tied to a particular sentence). During their school years, and particularly in adolescence, children also increase their ability to understand and to use figurative language (Nippold, 1993; Owens, 1984), that is, the creative use of words that make up puns, idioms, similes, metaphors, proverbs or sayings, sarcasm, and sometimes the punch lines of jokes.

What Is Syntax?

Not all languages rely heavily on word ordering to relay meaning, but the English language does (Tager-Flusberg, 1985). *Syntax* refers to the ordering of words in such a way that they can be understood. Grammatical rules tell us what the appropriate word orderings are for our intended meaning. The sentence "Jennifer visited Susie" does not carry the same meaning as "Susie visited Jennifer" because of the word ordering. Similarly, the words "Mouse the played catnip cat the with" carry no meaning in that order, but they are meaningful if rearranged into "The cat played with the catnip mouse."

Rules also tell us how to transform one sentence construction into another so that compound sentences, negatives, questions, passives, imperatives, and complex sentences with embedded (relative, adverbial, or nominal) clauses can be produced. As children advance through school, they learn to understand and to produce more complex sentences. For example, children do not fully understand the passive voice until approximately 11 to 13 years of age (Horgan, 1978). During adolescence, small but significant changes also occur in the length of both oral and written sentences with the increased use of (1) subordinate phrases and clauses and (2) cohesive conjunctions, such as *although, anyway, moreover, furthermore,* and *therefore* (Nippold, 1993).

What Is Morphology?

Morphology is one aspect of syntax. Some authors only enumerate four dimensions of language (semantics, syntax, pragmatics, and phonology), subsuming morphology under syntax.

Morphology deals with the prefixes and suffixes that are added to words in order to change meaning. Examples include: plurals to indicate number ("chair" versus "chairs"), verb tenses to express time ("laugh" versus "laugh*ed*"), markers to indicate possession ("girl" versus "girl*'s*"), *-er* and *-est* to indicate comparative and superlative adjectives ("pretty" versus "pretti*er*" versus "pretti*est*"), and markers to change one part of speech to another (as from an adjective to a noun, e.g., "lonely" to "loneli*ness*"). These prefixes and suffixes are referred to as *affixes* or *inflections* by some authors. The resulting words containing affixes are referred to as *inflectional forms*.

A morpheme is the smallest unit of meaning in a language. There are both bound and free morphemes. A free morpheme may be used alone, whereas a bound morpheme must be attached to a free morpheme in order to have meaning. All words are composed of at least one free morpheme; some words may have one or more bound morphemes attached to the free morpheme. For example, the word "friend" is composed of one free morpheme that has meaning. One or more bound morphemes may be added, making "friend*ly*," "*un*friend*ly*," "friend*less*," "friend*liness*," "friend*ship*," and "friend*lier*." There are rules for combining morphemes into words that must be followed (e.g., '*disfriend*" is not an allowable word and thus has no meaning).

What Is Pragmatics?

Pragmatics refers to the use of language in a social context for a particular purpose. The emphasis on pragmatics has been relatively recent in comparison to the attention paid to other components of language. However, its importance should not be underestimated, especially for school-age children. In fact, pragmatics has been called the area of most important language growth during both the school-age and adult years (Owens, 1984).

In order to maximally use language, children must learn how to initiate a conversation, take turns in conversation, maintain a conversational topic, change conversational topics, and close a conversation. Additionally, they must learn how to address different people by modifying their language. For example, research has shown that children as young as 4 years of age simplify their language when talking to younger children. Learning how to talk in different situations is also important. For example, children demonstrate knowledge of pragmatics if their language use differs when talking informally to the principal at a football game versus talking to the principal when being disciplined. Language can be used to request, inform, comment, warn, threaten, and promise (Newhoff & Leonard, 1983). Children must learn to phrase all of these uses politely and tactfully. One form of polite construction is the indirect request in which speakers pursue what they want in a roundabout manner. Children may comment, "That sure looks like fun" to someone playing with a videogame, as a hint to the other child to offer them a turn. Indirect requests are first learned in the preschool years (Owens, 1984) and continue to be refined in later years.

Another important pragmatic aspect of language is the ability of children to use language to gain entry into and maintain their position in a peer group. They do so by their ability to use current slang expressions and to employ other strategies to get along with their peers (Nippold, 1993). The slang expressions used differ by gender. Girls are more knowledgeable about slang expressions that refer to clothes and unpopular people, while boys tend to know more expressions for vehicles and money (Nippold, 1993).

What Are the Characteristics of a Language Disability?

The range of severity in language disabilities varies from mild to severe. Teachers will recognize that some children entering kindergarten are in need of help, whereas other children, due to the subtleties of their problems, may not be identified as language disabled until upper elementary, junior high, or even high school. School systems should adopt screening policies and procedures; and teachers, counselors, and other school personnel should learn to recognize subtle as well as obvious characteristics of language disabilities. Subtle problems may only be obvious when children meet with difficult situations, such as with difficult academic materials. Hayes, Norris, and Flaitz (1998) have even found that the academic performances of some children thought to be underachieving gifted adolescents may not be due to laziness but to subtle language disabilities that contrast with their overall abilities.

Some children who enter kindergarten with a history of language problems will have an IEP either from the school's preschool program or another preschool agency or from a conference held in the spring or summer to plan intervention during the kindergarten year. These children, in general, were slow in producing their first words or word combinations/sentences and continue to have grammatical errors, such as omitting "is"; omitting the articles "the", "a", and "an"; and using "me, him, her, them" for "I, he, she, they." They frequently need more time and make more errors in identifying pictures. They often have phonological errors as well. Olswang, Rodriguez, and Timler (1998) concluded from a review of the literature that most of these children show no delays in the cognitive, emotional, or sensory areas and that they develop language skills that are considered within normal limits during the first years of school. However, they noted that those who have a family history of either their parents or siblings having a learning disability or language disability were more at risk for not developing normal language. Contrastingly, Schuele and Hadley (1999) found literature that suggested that 50–70 percent of children with SLI do not "outgrow" their disability unless it is an expressive disability only, and then 50 percent or more catch up to their peers before entering kindergarten.

Kindergartners with obvious problems may not be able to follow oral directions, count correctly, name the days of the week, match sounds to letters, or sit still long enough to participate in learning experiences. Such children may be called slow, inattentive, impulsive, or obstinate (Wiig, 1986). As language concepts build on each other throughout the school years, these children may lag further and further behind. For example, children who do not grasp the concepts of "more" and "less" in a language arts workbook are apt to have more difficulty than their peers when introduced to "greater than" and "less than" in mathematics. As children pass from grade to grade, instruction becomes more abstract, with less use of manipulative items and concrete experiences. For example, mathematics lessons in the lower grades frequently involve manipulative tasks or pictures of items that can be checked off with a pencil as a child counts them. In the middle elementary grades these experiences become fewer and fewer, requiring that a child deal with more abstractions.

The remainder of this section will deal with typical problems that are associated with each of the dimensions of language. Remember that language behaviors are not always handily categorized into one of the dimensions and that the behaviors discussed are just some of the typical ones. As a teacher, you will need to further explore language disabilities. We urge you to consider taking courses in learning disabilities and language disabilities, and to learn independently from the many books available. Ask your speech-language pathologist for suggestions, look in educational catalogs, or examine the textbooks in the speech-language pathology section of a college bookstore. Also ask your administrator to consider an in-service on language development and language disabilities.

Semantics and Language Disabilities

Children with language disabilities have smaller vocabularies and so frequently give one-word answers and use fewer words to express themselves in comparison to their peers. This may mean that they communicate fewer concepts, and what they do communicate, they may communicate less effectively. Word finding or word retrieval problems are common. Even when a child has demonstrated the ability to use a word, he or she may have difficulty recalling it in a practical situation and, instead, may substitute nonspecific words or phrases, such as "stuff," "things," or "you know" for the appropriate word. Older children may substitute a definition of a word for the word itself (e.g., "the thing that you move to get water" for "faucet") or substitute a similar sounding word (e.g., "mural" for "moral"). The fillers that we all use, such as "uh," "um," and "okay," may be used with more frequency. Word and phrase repetitions may also be more prevalent. When asked to define words, children with language disabilities are apt to use functional definitions, such as "an apple is something that you can eat" (versus "fruit"); to change the subject; or to use fillers and word repetitions. Such children may also have difficulty understanding words because they have a smaller receptive vocabulary.

Words with multiple meanings typically prove to be perplexing problems that are compounded when the multiple meanings involve more than one part of speech. For example, a child may have difficulty expanding his or her meaning of the noun "family" to include not only the basic unit in society, but also a family of related plants or animals, a unit of a crime syndicate, and the first family of the United States. A word that can be used as different parts of speech, such as a noun or verb, is even more confusing. For example, every child is familiar with the four-legged barking creature that we call a "dog." However, to expand the meaning of the word "dog" and to understand it in the contexts of "you lucky dog," "don't dog my every step," "dog in the manger," "go to the dogs," "put on the dog," "he's a dog," or "my dogs are killing me" may simply not be possible for the language-disabled child without a good deal of help. Other examples should come to mind. Most people would probably agree that the word "draw" is a fairly simple word, but *Webster's Beginning Dictionary* (1980), written for students in the elementary grades, lists 16 definitions of the word "draw" as a verb and 4 as a noun, for a total of 20 different definitions. Moreover, there are the phrases "draw on," "draw out," "draw up," "draw aside," "draw forth," "draw in," "draw near," "draw back," and "draw the line." Not such a simple word after all. In the same dictionary, "set" has 14 definitions as a verb, 4 as an adjective, and 7 as a noun. One of these definitions, "a collection of mathematical elements," will certainly be important for comprehension in mathematics. Some difficulties with sentence comprehension may be due to choosing the wrong definitions for some of the words within a sentence.

Wiig (1986) noted that children with language disabilities had "difficulties interpreting prepositional phrases of location (at), direction (through), or time (before, after)" (p. 345) and difficulties "interpreting sentences with cause-effect or conditional (when . . . then, if . . . then) relationships and those with conjunction of clauses" (p. 346). For example, "we had dinner after we went to the movies" would typically be misinterpreted to mean that dinner occurred first, followed by the movies. She also noted that language-disabled children had problems "interpreting sentences with terms of inclusion, such as many, some, or several, or of exclusion, such as none, neither . . . nor, or combinations of these (all . . . except)" (p. 346).

The problems are varied and wide in scope. Children with language disabilities may exhibit trouble with synonyms and antonyms, demonstrative pronouns ("this," "that," "these," "those"), correct use of personal pronouns ("her did it"), word endings, verb tenses (and maintaining uniformity of tense throughout the communication), adjectives that provide information about spatial relationships ("near," "far," etc.), and forms of the copula "to be." Bracken (1988) did an interesting study of 49 opposite pairs and found that in approximately 70 percent of them the positive pole was learned before the negative pole. The positive pole either represented "more" of the concept quality, for example, "big" versus "little," or contained the root word of the concept, as in "male" and "female." Based on these findings, he advised in general that instruction begins with the positive pole whether working with a concept of just two polar opposites or with a continuum, such as all, most, several, few, and none. Exceptions to this rule included on-off, in front of-behind, large-small, thick-thin, all-none, early-late, always-never, over-under, forward-backward, rising-falling, healthy-sick, into-out, and arriving-leaving.

Young elementary children have fun with words, having "opposite days," when saying to someone "I hate you" means "I like you." Older children develop their own slang. At neither age are children with language disabilities able to understand and appropriately use what to them must seem a strange and confusing vocabulary. This causes their peers to laugh at and ostracize them from the group or, at the very least, to ignore them.

Figurative language refers to the creative use of language. Understanding figurative language in the forms of idioms, proverbs, metaphors, similes, sarcasm, or jokes may be especially difficult for children with language disabilities. Generally they have difficulty not only recognizing that figurative language should not be interpreted literally but also interpreting it (Seidenberg & Bernstein, 1986). To get a sense of the difficulties that these children encounter, consider the following handful of idioms and think about the difficulty that a child would have making sense of whatever context they were in if he or she chose the literal interpretation:

- raining cats and dogs
- toe the line
- all thumbs
- butterflies in your stomach
- hit the roof
- burn one's fingers
- read between the lines
- watched pot never boils
- puppy love
- kick the bucket

- hit the hay
- hang loose
- bury the hatchet
- pulling my leg
- forty winks
- rub the wrong way
- crack me up
- throw a party
- hold your tongue
- bite off more than you can chew
- bull-headed
- keep a straight face
- yellow streak down his back
- green with envy
- head and shoulders above the rest

Now consider a scenario that was overheard during a carpool of four sixth- and seventh-graders. "Amy" and "Josh" had been fussing at each other, and finally Amy burst out with, "You're not being nice; you just don't like me." Josh responded. "I do so like you. Just the other day, I stood up for you. Somebody said you weren't fit to eat with the pigs, and I said you were." Poor Amy, who had difficulty with language, never understood the slap in the face (pardon my idiom). Just how early children understand figurative meanings is debatable. One variable affecting children's understanding may be their exposure to various experiences. For example, Abkarian, Jones, and West (1992) gave the example of "skating on thin ice" and hypothesized that the child who has experienced ice skating on ponds where ice is sometimes thin might be more able to understand this idiom. They also point out that children's experiences are often tied to their socioeconomic status. Qualls and Harris (1999) found that geographical location, social cultures, and frequency of use also played a role in which idioms were understood.

Proverbs will also pose problems for the child with a language disability. Consider:

- A penny saved is a penny earned.
- Many hands make light work.
- An apple a day keeps the doctor away.
- Rome wasn't built in a day.
- Birds of a feather flock together.

Analogies, such as those frequently seen on achievement tests, are another potential source of problems—horse is to foal as dog is to puppy or inch is to foot as ounce is to pound. Analogies are frequently used in mathematics and science. Masterson and Perrey (1999) warn that the child with a language disability may not be able to learn from analogies used as instructional techniques. They provide suggestions and abbreviated lesson plans for teaching analogies (Masterson & Perry, 1994, 1999).

Similes ("quiet as a mouse"), homophones (words pronounced the same but spelled differently, such as "know" and "no"), homographs (words spelled the same with two different meanings, such as "bank" referring to a depository for money and the river bank), and heteronyms (two words spelled the same but pronounced differently with different meanings, such as "suspect" the noun and "suspect" the verb) also are often difficult. When reading, children are frequently expected to recognize the intended meaning of multiple-meaning words (homographs) quickly and accurately, especially if the teacher expects them to have been mastered in an earlier grade. In oral discourse, homophones have multiple meanings because the spelling cannot be seen and thus provides no clue. Children with language disabilities can easily become confused and lost, and the teacher may have no idea why.

Syntax and Language Disabilities

Problems in the ordering of words may be due to problems with ideation (the process of formulating one's thoughts) or syntax, or both. Details may be sequenced illogically.

A particular problem occurs with the transformation of sentences. This refers to changes (rearranging, deletions, and substitutions of words) that are made in the base structure of a sentence (such a sentence is a simple, declarative, affirmative sentence written in the active voice) in order to form new sentences. Sentences in which the usual order of words is changed present problems in expression as well as in comprehension. For example, the usual subject-verb-object order is changed in passive sentences, so that "Jason was beaten by Brian in Monopoly" would typically be misinterpreted as subject (Jason)-verb (beat)-object (Brian) or "Jason beat Brian." Sentences that contain both a direct object and an indirect object are also sometimes difficult to interpret. Children with language disabilities may interpret "Susan showed Mary the monkey" as "Susan showed Mary to the monkey."

Difficulty with "wh" questions (what, why, who, when, which, where, whose) may also be displayed. For example, a child may give a "what" answer to a "why" question (Simon, 1979). "Wh" questions are more difficult to answer when the question refers to events, objects, or people outside of the immediate situation (Parnell, Amerman, & Harting, 1986). Furthermore, ability to ask "wh" questions enables children to learn about the world around them (Schwabe, Olswang, & Kriegsmann, 1986), whether it is the 2-year-old asking why or the school-age child who did not understand the directions for an assignment.

Other problems are created with ambiguous sentences, such as "teasing friends can get you into trouble." The child with a language disability might not consider the two possible interpretations: (1) the act of teasing friends may get you into trouble, and (2) friends who tease you may cause you to do something to get into trouble.

In English grammar lessons, children with language disabilities have trouble making up sentences using a particular sentence structure, especially if the sentence is complex. Their sentences tend to be short and lack the syntactical complexity afforded by coordinate and subordinate conjunctions and embedded phrases. For vocabulary lessons, sentences that are formed from the vocabulary words tend to be short, simple, and agrammatical (Wiig, 1986).

Other difficulties include problems with reflexives (e.g., "myself," "herself," "themselves"); the omission of "to" in infinitives; irregular past-tense verbs, irregular plural nouns, and difficulties with auxiliary verbs. Words in a sentence may be slurred and run together. Beginning a sentence with "Um, uh, last night, well on yesterday . . . ." is referred to as a *false start*. This is a common problem related to the ability to order thoughts and words and to think of the right words. The difficulties that children with language disabilities show in repeating, formulating, and comprehending more complex sentences generally represent delays that follow the pattern of normal syntactic development (Wigg, 1986).

Morphology and Language Disabilities

Children with language disabilities frequently ignore word endings, such as plural suffixes, comparative and superlative adjective suffixes, the -*ly* endings of adverbs, and low stress words such as prepositions and conjunctions (Wiig, 1986). Difficulties occur with possessives, the past tense of verbs, and prefixes.

The inability of children with language disabilities to comprehend and use derived words, such as "loveliness" from "lovely," implies that "they do not learn the word formation rules (morphology) at the same rate and with the same consistency and degree of sophistication [as their peers] with normal language development" (Wigg, 1986, pp. 346–347).

Pragmatics and Language Disabilities

Children with language disabilities frequently do not give considerations to who the listener is, the age of the listener, the degree of formality of the situation or environment, the amount of time that they have to convey their messages, and how well they know the listener. These children often use a simpler, more informal style of communication with everyone (Wigg, 1986). They may maintain poor eye contact, infringe on their conversational partner's turn to speak, and fail to maintain an appropriate distance between themselves and their conversational partner.

Children who have difficulty with pragmatics may not consider the listener's verbal and nonverbal responses or the listener's ability to follow the speaker's train of thought. In contrast, effective speakers make note of the listener's responses, attempt to interpret those responses, and, if necessary, change their communication strategies. Consider the following mental scenarios that a speaker faced with a frowning listener might engage in:

Possible problem: Did the listener hear?

Possible solution: Repeat the message loudly.

Possible problem: Did the listener understand the meaning?

Possible solution: Rephrase the message.

Possible problem: Is the listener unhappy, disapproving?

Possible solutions: Provide supporting reasons or temper the message to go along with what the listener evidently feels.

Possible problem: Was the topic of conversation switched without giving the listener any warning?

Possible solution: Inform the listener that the speaker's train of thought changed.

A few other listener reactions include edging away from the speaker, smiling, nodding, laughing, and other emotional responses like crying or swearing.

An effective communicator is capable of planning strategies ahead of time. A child who knows he or she is going to be in trouble for a misdeed may plan whether to accept responsibility, to offer an excuse, or to blame another child. Older youth and adults plan how to answer anticipated questions in a job interview. Effective communicators can also change strategies when they recognize that the one being used is not working out well. As children mature, they learn how to negotiate and persuade, how to choose words and tone of voice, and how to appropriately modulate volume and rate of speech.

People with language disabilities tend not to couch their speech in polite terms or to show consideration for others in their language use. For example, they may make demands (imperative statements), such as "Turn off the radio," instead of requests, such as "Will you turn off the radio, please?" or indirect requests, such as "My head hurts" (hint: the radio is causing the headache), or "Are you still listening to the radio?" (hint: the radio is bothering me).

Unfortunately, when children with language disabilities have difficulty comprehending language, they tend not to ask clarifying questions or to indicate that they did not understand and need help. Thus, they may not respond at all or may respond inappropriately. Obviously, this behavior leads to academic problems. Perhaps less obviously, it leads to social problems.

What Sort of Assessment Is There for Language?

Deciding if a particular child's language problem requires remediation is not always easy. As with all task performance, variability occurs across "normal" children and within the same "normal" child. In other words, there is a wide range of behaviors that can be considered normal. Each school district will have criteria that help to make this decision. One problem that arises is that criteria vary from school district to school district.

There are also personal characteristics that affect language. When making referrals and when choosing and interpreting diagnostic procedures, a speech-language pathologist and other concerned school personnel should be careful to consider the effects of the following factors on language:

- Ethnic Background: How an adult approaches a child may affect a child's performance. For example, black and Hispanic children tend to score better when they are familiar with the tester. Therefore, the tester should engage in informal play with a younger child and in verbal interaction with an older one before beginning to test (Adler, 1990).
- Socioeconomic Status (SES): Parental education, occupational status, and income are closely associated with SES. Because these factors are reflected in language, they must be considered in evaluating a child's linguistic functioning.
- Bilingualism: Just as not all languages contain the same speech sounds, not all languages follow the same rules. The bilingual child has some facility in two or more distinct languages. This is further discussed later in this chapter.
- Use of Nonstandard English Dialects: Dialects, such as African American English, Southern White Nonstandard English, and Appalachian, follow many of the rules of Standard American English but also have some different rules (Labov, 1972). Note that these dialects are referred to as *non*standard and not *sub*standard. It is the position of the American Speech-Language-Hearing Association (ASHA) that no dialectical variation of English is a disorder of speech or language. Social dialects are rule-based and are not to be considered "less than" but only "different from" that which is recognized as standard English. This, too, is further discussed later in this chapter.

Assessment is initiated either through routine screening procedures or through referrals. On a referral form and/or behavior checklist, a teacher will have alerted the speech-language pathologist to any particular areas of language that are causing a child academic or social difficulties. Particular attention in assessment can then be given to these areas.

Screening

It has been suggested that every child entering elementary school be screened for language disabilities. Others who should be screened include children who have been referred for possible language problems; children at risk for language problems; children who are having difficulty learning to read, spell, and write; and children who are at critical educational transitions, such as those moving from elementary school to junior high or moving from junior high to high school (Wigg & Semel, 1984).

Evaluation and Diagnosis

What children can do and what they cannot do are both important; assumptions should not be made about either. The purpose of an evaluation is to describe a child's language status and, if a problem does exist, to determine goals that can be recommended to the IEP committee and potential remedial procedures for reaching those goals.

To begin with, a hearing evaluation should be conducted because hearing losses may affect language comprehension and production. Then standardized norm-referenced tests or informal testing procedures, or both, may be used in a diagnostic assessment. In addition to language, some standardized tests also examine memory, the ability to sequence, and auditory processing (the ability to understand oral language in the absence of a peripheral hearing loss; also called *central auditory processing*, it takes place in the brain). One informal testing procedure is the spontaneous language sample, which is probably the "most useful approach to examination of older children" (Newhoff & Leonard, 1983). A language sample involves recording the language that a child uses in a particular situation. The situation should be arranged so that a representative sample can be obtained. For example, if the goal were to obtain the best language performance that a child was capable of in an informal play situation, then the child should be relaxed and comfortable. (Labov, 1972, has recommended that because less privileged children may feel threatened in a formal diagnostic situation with an unfamiliar adult, even if a play situation is being simulated, a more informal situation, perhaps on the floor with at least one other peer, would create a situation in which such children would talk more freely.)

Sometimes a child may be able to help isolate difficulties if questions focusing on each dimension of language are asked. For example, when probing for problems in the area of semantics, a speech-language pathologist might ask children if they notice whether they have difficulty thinking of the right word to use (Wigg & Semel, 1984). It should be noted that in an assessment it is not always a simple matter to separate the components of language (Newhoff & Leonard, 1983).

The language assessment is certainly not complete without information about a child's cognitive status. The school psychologist and a child's teacher would have valuable input in this area. Researchers disagree on the exact nature of the relationship between cognition and language, but they do agree that there is a relationship. More and more of the literature in speech-language pathology is taking exception with how the cognitive hypothesis has been used to determine who is and who is not eligible for language therapy. Because the cognitive hypothesis states that cognitive development is necessary for language development, those children whose language abilities are at the level expected based on their cognitive development are often ineligible for language therapy. Only if their language abilities are less than expected based on their IQ tests are children declared eligible for language therapy. The argument against this is that there are factors other than cognitive ability that affect language. These factors include environmental and nurturing factors. Furthermore, language gains in therapy have been made with mentally handicapped children whose language age was above their mental age yet below their chronological age (Casby, 1992; Cole, Coggins, & Vanderstoep, 1999; Cole, Mills, & Kelley, 1994). Cole et al. (1994) recommend that the IEP committee look at the child's unmet communicative needs in their decision-making process.

What about the Language Abilities of Students Who Speak Dialects or English as a Second Language?

As noted in Chapter 2, Standard American English (SAE) is the language used by the media, the government, and most businesses. (Refer back to Chapter 2 for definitions of dialect, English as a second language, and limited English proficiency.) The number of children who come to school speaking something other than SAE is increasing and is projected to continue to do so. The problem is especially difficult in inner cities and in certain states. For example, the student population in California speaks over 130 languages (Goldberg, 1997). Many have probably never even heard of some of the languages that are spoken by students, such as Chamorro, which is spoken in Guam. Also, as noted in Chapter 2, many believe that the first language or dialect should be preserved so the child may better identify with the family and community who speak the first language or dialect.

Politics has entered the fray, and legislation has been passed mandating how education should address this issue. Arguments have been presented for teaching children their first language as well as English as a second language. Their first language is taught so that they have a good cognitive linguistic base from which to learn both the academic curriculum as well as English. If a dialect of SAE is spoken, then bidialectical education is used. Schools that follow this reasoning must then address the issue of how long bilingual or bidialectical education should continue. Other schools believe in an English immersion program in which the curriculum is presented in SAE only.

Often a child who is struggling to learn SAE and struggling with the academic curriculum is referred to the speech-language pathologist for a language evaluation. Again, if the speech-language pathologist is not proficient in that child's language or dialect, someone (such as someone else in the school system, a parent, or a community member) must be found who can translate and provide information about that language or dialect. The speech-language pathologist will conduct the language evaluation in the first language as well as in SAE. In striving not to over- or underidentify children with language disabilities, two problems arise: (1) a lack of formal assessments and norms in the first language or dialect and (2) a lack of bias-free, formal assessments for non-SAE speakers in SAE (Rhyner, Kelly, Brantley, & Krueger, 1999). Sometimes local norms can be established, or modifications of standardized tests devised (Washington & Craig, 1999). Testing may also be complicated by cultural differences. For example, differences in nonverbal communication, such as the way a child has been taught to interact and converse with adults (which, of course, includes teachers), if not understood, may affect decisions about the child's language status. The teacher may be asked to provide information about the degree of opportunity a child has for interacting with English speakers and the amount of interaction that the child chooses to participate in when an opportunity is present (for example, at recess). Another problem that may arise is communicating with the child's parents. Federal law mandates that information conveyed to parents be presented in their preferred language, which may again necessitate an interpreter.

How are the results of a language evaluation interpreted for children with non-SAE backgrounds? For the child who speaks a dialect, the term *speech-language difference* is used when the child appropriately uses the rules of a dialect. In other words, there is only a difference, not a disorder. For the child who speaks English as a second language, the child's performance on the native language evaluation is the key. If a child does not have a language disorder in the first language, then whatever problems are present in SAE are assumed to be due just to the fact that the child is still learning SAE. A language disorder is present only if there is a disorder in both languages. Roseberry-McKibbon (1994) cautions that there are several types of errors that occur during second language learning that are normal and should neither be the basis of an evaluation to determine if there is a language disorder nor be considered as representing a language disorder. Some of these typical errors include:

- Silent Period: Learning a second language may begin with a silent period during which the speaker presumably focuses on understanding rather than on talking.
- Interlanguage Codeswitching: The child goes back and forth between the two languages or dialects (the term *codeswitching* is also sometimes used to refer to the ability to change communicative style depending on the audience and/or situation, i.e., talking to the principal on the playground versus talking to the principal in the office when in trouble or talking to a playmate versus an adult).
- Interference: The child puts English words in the order that would be correct in the first language, such as placing an adjective after the noun (as would occur in Spanish) rather than before the noun (as would occur in English).
- Fossilization: A child just seems to continue to use some errors no matter what.

Following are some of the language rule differences between dialects used in the United States and SAE. First, in African American English, look for:

- Copula deletion in sentences, such as "the paper on the desk" for "the paper is on the desk"
- Use of singular verb in present tense, third person, such as "he play" for "he plays"
- Use of "a" (versus "an") regardless of the initial sound of the following word
- Use of "is" with all persons and numbers in the present tense, such as "I is," "you (singular) is," "he is," "she is," "it is," "we is," "you (plural) is," and "they is"
- Deletion of the plural marker, such as "two coat" for "two coats"
- Addition of a plural marker, such as "childrens" for "children" or "that mines"
- Use of "hisself" for the reflexive pronoun "himself"
- Use of multiple negatives, such as "I don't never want no dog" (number of negatives may indicate strength of negation)
- Use of objective pronouns as subjects, such as "him" for "he"

- Deletion of possessive marker, such as "Mary cookie" for "Mary's cookie"
- Substituting a noun and comment for a noun and verb, such as "My sister, she smart" for "My sister is smart"

In Southern White English, the following differences are common:

- Double modals, such as "I might could be fixing to"
- Deletion of relative pronouns, such as "the dog bit me" for "the dog that bit me"
- Use of double negatives
- Use of objective pronouns as subjects, such as "him" for "he"

Some characteristics of the Appalachian dialect include:

- Double modals
- Deletion of relative pronouns
- Use of "hisself" for the reflexive pronoun "himself"
- Addition of a plural marker
- Use of "his'n" for "his"

What Effect Does a Language Disability Have on Academic Performance?

Children with language disabilities are at high risk of failing academically, as the reader will already have deduced from the examples given of problems that children with language disabilities have. Children who do not have a command of oral language will have difficulty learning to read and write. Think about beginning reading experiences. Textbook companies make use of the fact that stories about experiences that are familiar to children are the easiest for children to understand and to learn to read. However, children with language disabilities may be unable to organize experiences in their own minds. When a teacher asks children with language disabilities, "What do you think happened next?" or gives them a worksheet with pictures or sentences to order into a story, even if the children have experienced the events in the story, they may be unable to organize and order the events.

Another approach to reading involves asking kindergarten or first-grade children to dictate sentences about pictures that they have drawn. After the teacher prints the sentences under the pictures, the children are asked to "read" the sentences. The child with a language disability may find it difficult to dictate a sentence, especially a sentence without errors, and then may have a difficult time "reading" the sentence and including any corrections that the teacher may have made. For example, auxiliary verbs, even when added, may continue to be omitted in the "reading."

A definite connection has been made between dyslexia (a type of learning disability that involves problems in reading, spelling, and writing) and specific language impairment, especially if the children also have poor auditory memories and short attention spans. Problems will also arise in mathematics, partly due to the exactness of the vocabulary and partly due to the need to carefully manipulate language, especially in story problems (Simon, 1979).

As a heavier emphasis is placed on social studies, science, literature, and other subjects, basic skills in reading and mathematics do not continue to be taught as they were in lower grades. Children are expected to use those basic skills to learn to reason, to prepare written and oral reports, and to analyze stories in terms of character and plot development. What is automatic for normally developing youngsters is still difficult for children who have language disabilities, and they are left further and further behind.

Catts (1997) suggests that children who will have difficulty learning to read can be identified before they actually fail at reading. He has designed a checklist to be used with children at the end of kindergarten or the beginning of first grade. He cautions that no one item can conclusively identify a child who will have difficulty; however, the more items checked, the greater the likelihood for reading difficulties. This checklist can be found in his article and can be photocopied for professional use.

Is There a Relationship Between Language Disabilities and ADHD?

Attention deficit hyperactivity disorder (ADHD) is diagnosed by a physician based on observational data. It rarely exists by itself but is generally accompanied by problems in language, literacy, and social/emotional adjustment (Westby, 1999). In the past, ADHD has been considered a disorder of attention; the current view of ADHD holds that it is a disorder of behavioral inhibition. When behavior cannot be inhibited through internalized rules and consequences, the characteristic inattention, impulsivity, and hyperactivity are seen. It is the most prevalent childhood psychiatric disorder, affecting as many as 3 to 5 percent of our school-age children. Somewhere between 20 and 60 percent of the children with ADHD are apt to also have language disabilities (Oram, Fine, Okamoto, & Tannock, 1999). These language disabilities are especially noticeable in the child's difficulty with maintenance of a topic, sequencing events, comprehension, and socializing. A child who has a language disability along with ADHD will qualify for communication services under IDEA. If ADHD is the only diagnosis, a child may qualify for services under Section 504 of the Rehabilitation Act of 1973, as amended.

Does a Language Disability Affect Psychological and Sociological Adjustment?

Yes, those with language disabilities are at risk for developing psychological and social problems. Language is the primary avenue used in developing interpersonal relationships, including friendships and the ability to become part of a group. Their facility with language affects whether they are accepted into a group or ostracized by their peers (Reed, McLeod, & McAllister, 1999). Two studies (Hadley & Rice, 1991; Rice, Sell, & Hadley, 1991) found that children as young as preschool age had some awareness of their own communication abilities as well as those of others and preferred to play with communicatively responsive peers. An interesting consequence of this is that children who do not interact as much with other children do not get as many chances to hone their language skills.

Although many factors may contribute to social problems, children with language disabilities have been rated by teachers as having a variety of social problems (Fujiki, Brinton, Morgan, & Hart, 1999). These children may need guidance from their teachers and referrals by their teachers to guidance counselors or student advisors who can help them as well as having goals dealing with pragmatics written into their IEPs.

Mack and Warr-Leeper (1992) noted that boys with chronic behavior disorder exhibited a much higher prevalence of language disabilities than would be expected. They suggested that because language is the basis for establishing and maintaining social relationships, their difficulties with language contributed to the social and emotional problems.

Many postulate that severe communicative incompetence may be the underlying basis for misbehaviors like hitting, biting, temper tantrums, and destroying whatever is within reach. It has also been suggested that such behaviors may be communicative attempts, such as "I do not want to _____" or "I want _____," and that when the child is given a more appropriate sign for whatever the communicative attempt is and then is appropriately reinforced for using that sign, the disruptive behaviors decrease. Johnson and Reichle (1993) recommend looking for antecedents to the challenging behaviors in order to identify what the communicative intent might have been, and then they suggest interventions that can be used to try to stop the challenging behaviors.

What about Remediation?

The individualized educational program (IEP), drawn up with the parents after a complete assessment takes place, will provide the goals and guidelines for remediation. A team effort is definitely needed. Potentially the classroom teacher, a speech-language pathologist, a reading specialist, and other special education personnel may all work with a child. Each needs to know what the others are doing and why. Their efforts need to be coordinated.

Goals in the IEP will frequently be stated in percentages. For example, if a child uses appropriate verb tenses 40 percent of the time, then the goal might be that the child, by a certain date, would demonstrate 80 percent accurate use. In order to stimulate carryover of any behavior, a child needs to understand the purpose of what he or she is learning and to produce the behavior easily many times in situations that are as meaningful as possible (Simon, 1979). Cooperative parents might be asked to provide structured generalization or carryover experiences.

Wilson, Lanza, and Barton (1988) have suggested that children with language disabilities may need help developing thinking skills. They used Bloom's taxonomy of thinking levels (knowledge, comprehension, application, analysis, synthesis, and evaluation) to identify strategies for helping children increase the variety and complexity of their thinking skills. For example, they recommended that children be encouraged to (1) recognize and recall facts from a story or experience; (2) relate the facts in order; (3) explain ideas; (4) relate the experience or story to their own lives or knowledge of others' experiences; (5) compare and contrast events in the story to each other or to personal experiences; (6) create new parts to a story; (7) identify logical next events; and (8) make judgments, such as was it a good idea for the characters to act as they did.

A teacher's ability to teach coping skills is only limited by lack of knowledge of what havoc a language disability can cause in a child's academic progress and the teacher's creativity. For example, Ukrainetz (1998) helped students learn to draw stick figures as a notational system. When developing a story, children with language disabilities have difficulty thinking of what to say, logically sequencing the story, moving the story forward, and remembering where they are in their telling of the story. If they have to worry about writing as they do all of this, scanning back through their story to see where they are, et cetera, the problem is compounded. By using stick-figure drawings, they can outline their story more quickly and "read" their notes more easily. This technique can be used for either oral or written assignments. Time saved by the child may be devoted to an additional goal on the assignment, such as vocabulary development with a dictionary or thesaurus or learning to insert sequencing words, such as *first, then, next,* and *last,* into their stories. Students have also been taught to use the stick-figure drawings to improve their listening comprehension and note taking.

Teaching techniques can be adapted to identified problem areas, perhaps with the help of a teacher's aide or parent volunteer. For example, a child with a language disability will have difficulty with scrambled sentences. You might as well ask some of these children to climb Mt. McKinley as to take a series of unrelated words and reorganize them into a proper sentence. This child just does not know where to start. How can they learn? One way is to provide them with a book that is just below their reading ability (so that the task is not compounded with reading difficulties), ask them to go through and make a list of every first word in all of the sentences until there is a list of 40 or so, then discuss the most frequent first word, the similarities of the rest, and so on. It will be surprising how many will catch on and not cringe at the sight of the next page of scrambled sentences.

Teachers might also consider giving more attention to explaining and teaching humor, slang, and the unusual uses of language found in idioms, similes, irony, and proverbs. Perhaps a unit could be developed with an art teacher in which idioms are drawn in two ways, the literal and the figurative. A list of all the similes found in a social studies textbook or a book used for reading (you'll find more than you expected) could be kept on a bulletin board and reviewed at odd moments, such as when there are 3 minutes before lunch time. Books like Shel Silverstein's *Light in the Attic*, Peggy Parish's Amelia Bedelia books, or *The True Story of the Three Little Pigs by A. Wolf* could either be read to the children or be used as part of the reading curriculum. Spector (1992) provides a detailed explanation with examples of the various ways in which jokes are humorous. For example, a whole word is confused with a larger word that contains the whole word in question, as in the joke: What <u>pet</u> makes the best music? A trum<u>pet</u>. Word ambiguities, two words that vary by only one phoneme, word reversals, changes in syllable or word stress, and misinterpretations of words with more than one definition are just some of the humor techniques that are explained. Teachers could use the information in his article as a way to teach humor to children with language difficulties. The children could learn and practice their knowledge through group activities, independent reports, or any other way that your creativity dictates. They might be rewarded with a chance to publish a joke column in the school newspaper including all of the jokes that they understand.

Teachers might also go to speech therapy with their students as well as consult with the speech-language pathologist to find out how to help their students with various problems. For example, naming or word-finding difficulties are frequent problems. The speech-language pathologist may have found that visual imagery helps with being able to recall the word sought as well as decreasing the time needed to recall it. When teachers also understand and use this strategy, the students benefit.

A teacher, or better yet the school as a whole, could strive to find adults with language disabilities who are successful and could serve as mentors either in or out of the classroom. These mentors could (1) offer insights into coping strategies and hints on how to pay better attention during critical times, such as when the teacher is giving instructions, and (2) discuss emotions and social problems, letting the child know that others have been faced with similar problems, have coped, and made it. A mentor who is not available during school hours could be a pen pal on the internet, and the e-mail going back and forth could be used as a reading comprehension and/or writing assignment.

When selecting textbooks, teachers should consider the language difficulty of textbooks in relationship to the language proficiencies of the children they have, or expect to have, in their classrooms. Teachers should analyze their own discourse in relationship to the language proficiencies of their charges. Teachers' rate of presentation, complexity of sentence structure (syntax), use of vocabulary (will it be understood by the children?), interaction between syntax and vocabulary, length of explanation or direction, and use of visual (body language or seeing the item being discussed) and tactile (feeling the item being discussed) clues should conform to the children's abilities. Teachers can also help by rephrasing their messages rather than simply repeating what they have said; using concrete, direct wording rather than abstractions or subtleties; using nonverbal clues along with verbal messages; asking children to demonstrate nonverbally (pointing, doing what they were told, etc.) that they have understood a message; providing visual examples of what they are talking about; encouraging children to indicate that they do not understand and to ask clarifying questions; and never assuming that children understand.

Adolescents who have language problems are attracting increased, well-deserved, and long-overdue attention. Typically these youth have gotten lost in the cracks of the educational system, and in many states and school districts they still do get lost. It has been common to find that children who received language services in elementary school no longer receive services when they move on to junior (or middle) and senior high schools. These students still have the same needs, no matter which grade they are in, and their continued need is being increasingly recognized. Part of the blame for these students not being served for the language needs may lie in the fact that the traditional pullout model has been typically used as the service delivery model. Secondary teachers are more apt to object to their students being pulled out; the students are also more apt to object to missing their classes. When other service delivery models have been implemented, results have been very favorable. Those that have been found to work best include (1) the collaborative consultation model, in which the speech-language pathologist collaborates with the student's teachers to provide extra language help, and (2) the self-contained program, in which language remediation is offered by the speech-language pathologist as a course (Larson & McKinley, 1993; Larson, McKinley, & Boley, 1993; Work, Cline, Ehren, Keiser, & Wujek, 1993). It has even been reported that the dropout rate for students with language disabilities decreases in both rural and urban schools when appropriate language remediation along with other special help and programs, such as vocational education, is provided (Larson, McKinley, & Boley, 1993).

What Does the Future Hold for Children and Youth with Language Disabilities?

Authorities are in general agreement that although some symptoms of language disabilities will change over time, others will continue into adulthood. Some adults avoid the linguistic situations with which they have the most difficulty. They may avoid new social situations because they are poor at conversations, having difficulty beginning conversations, maintaining topics, shifting topics, and ending conversations. Their coping strategies in the workplace may fail at least initially when they encounter new experiences, such as a new job, a new boss, or a promotion. However, it can be expected that adults who have been identified as having language disabilities and have received language therapy as youngsters are in a better position to cope as adults.

Case History

Jerrid

Jerrid was first seen as a 3-year-old. At that time he spoke very little, was difficult to understand, and had difficulties in all language areas. Today he is a third-grader.

The only speech sound errors he has are on the voiceless and voiced "th" sounds. However, he exhibits problems in all aspects of language and so has academic problems. With an IQ in the normal range, he qualifies for services as a child with a learning disability in language and for related services in communication (both articulation and language).

Typical language errors include:

- Subject–verb disagreement, e.g., "we was." This is even more difficult when the sentence starts with "there" and the noun that will determine whether a singular or plural verb is needed follows the verb in the sentence, e.g., "there are two birds."
- Adjective noun agreement, e.g., "a tools"
- Difficulty making explanations, e.g., Question: "What is a piano?" Answer: "Something that you sing, you're at the city, you sing it and it sounds good."
- Problems with prepositions, e.g., Question: "What are pockets?" Answer: "Put something on it, put something in it, like money."
- Omission of words, e.g., Instruction: "Tell me about a backpack." Answer: "If you don't bring back, you gotta stay in recess."
- Difficulty with semantics, e.g., calling a painter a "paint guy" and stating the function instead of naming the item.
- Comprehension, e.g., when looking at a picture book about a circus, having no idea what the sentence "The circus elephants circled the ring three times" meant because he was unable to conceive of "circled" as a verb rather than as a reference to the shape or of "ring" as anything besides jewelry that goes on a finger.

Unlike many children who have had so many language and academic problems, Jerrid continues to work hard and says he knows he has to do his best.

Summary

Some Important Points to Remember

- *Learning disabilities* refers to difficulties in listening, reading, reasoning, or mathematical skills.
- Emotional, hearing, and visual problems can coexist with a learning disability.
- Language delay is a subset of the larger problem of learning disability.
- The ability to learn language is most likely due to innate factors as well as the environment and nurturing.
- Language disabilities may be due to developmental or acquired factors.
- Most children with specific language impairment will also have articulation and/or phonology disorders.
- The cognitive hypothesis has been used to determine which children qualify for language therapy, but this may not be an appropriate criterion.

- Evaluations of children who are bidialectical or bilingual must take into consideration the rules of both dialects or languages.
- Semantics deals with the meanings words evoke.
- Syntax refers to the ordering of words.
- Morphology, an aspect of syntax, deals with prefixes and suffixes.
- A morpheme is the smallest meaningful unit in a language.
- Pragmatics refers to the use of language in a social context for a particular purpose.
- Parental education, occupation, and income are reflected in a child's linguistic functioning.
- There are standardized tests for assessing language ability.
- Language disabilities range from mild to severe.
- Children with language disabilities may have smaller vocabularies than their peers.
- Words with multiple meanings present particular problems for the semantically involved language-delayed child.
- Children with problems of syntax have difficulty in ordering words using a particular sentence structure.
- Children with morphological problems frequently ignore word endings.
- Children with problems of pragmatics often use a simpler style of communication than do their non language-disabled peers.
- Children with problems in pragmatics tend not to use polite terms or show consideration for their listeners.
- Children with language disabilities are at high risk of academic failure.
- There is a relationship between language disabilities and ADHD.
- Communication problems may be reflected in behavior problems.
- The effects of language disabilities in childhood are often observed in adulthood, but those who received speech-language therapy in childhood are better prepared to cope than those who did not.

"Do"s and "Don't"s for Teachers

"Do"s:

- Be alert to the presence of any children with language disabilities in the classroom.
- Be sure to understand the provisions of the IEP regarding your responsibilities.
- Refer children suspected of language delay to a speech-language pathologist.
- Recognize that children with oral language problems have difficulty communicating.

"Don't"s:

- Do not confuse sensory problems of hearing or vision with learning problems.
- Do not expect all languages to follow the same rules.

Self-Test

True or False:

1. Language disability and learning disability refer to the same condition. _____

2. Some language disorders show up as early as 18 months of age. _____

3. Language disability is identified by most authorities as a part of the learning disabilities picture. _____

4. Hearing impairment may cause a speech problem but not a language problem. _____

5. Language development has little, if anything, to do with social and cultural contexts. _____

6. The components of language include phonology. _____

7. Semantics is a component of language primarily focused on prefixes and suffixes of words. _____

8. Pragmatics is simply another term for morphology. _____

9. Language development is rule-based. _____

10. Parental occupation and education as well as income are factors to consider in the assessment of language. _____

11. Auditory processing is of little concern to one who makes assessment of language performance. _____

12. The teacher can make valuable contributions to the evaluation of a child's language status by making information available to the speech-language pathologist concerning the child's cognitive capabilities. _____

13. A language disability rarely retards the scholastic progress of a child. _____

14. Synonyms and antonyms are particularly troublesome for the language-disabled child whose primary problem is one of syntax. _____

15. Difficulties of repeating, comprehending, and formulating complex sentences are usually related to a problem with semantics. _____

16. Children who have problems with oral language usage will most likely have difficulties with reading and writing. _____

17. The suffix "ly" is an example of a free morpheme. _____

18. A language disorder may be present in the language learned second but not in the first or native language. _____

19. The teacher should refer to the speech-language pathologist any child suspected of having a language problem. _____

20. Head injuries may cause acquired language disabilities. _____

References

Adler, S. (1990). Multicultural clients: Implications for the SLP. *Language, Speech, and Hearing Services in Schools, 21*, 135–139.

ASHA Committee on Language. (1983). Definition of language. *ASHA, 25*(6), 44.

Bliss, L. S. (1987). "I can't talk anymore; my mouth doesn't want to." The development and clinical applications of modal auxiliaries. *Language, Speech, and Hearing Services in Schools, 18*, 72–79.

Bloom, L., & Lahey, M. (1978). *Language development and language disorders*. New York: Wiley.

Bracken, B. A. (1988). Rate and sequence of positive and negative poles in basic concept acquisition. *Language, Speech, and Hearing Services in Schools, 19*, 410–417.

Casby, M. W. (1992). The cognitive hypothesis and its influence on speech-language services in schools. *Language, Speech, and Hearing Services in Schools, 23*, 198–202.

Catts, H. W. (1997. The early identification of language-based reading disabilities. *Language, Speech, and Hearing Services in Schools, 28*, 86–87.

Cole, K. N., Coggins, T. E., & Vanderstoep, C. (1999). The influence of language-cognitive profile on discourse intervention outcome. *Language, Speech, and Hearing Services in Schools, 30*, 61–67.

Cole, K. N., Mills, P. E., & Kelley, D. (1994). Agreement of assessment profiles used in cognitive referencing. *ASHA, 25*, 25–31.

Fujiki, M., Brinton, B., Morgan, M., & Hart, C. H. (1999). Withdrawn and social behavior of children with language impairment. *Language, Speech, and Hearing Services in Schools, 30*, 183–195.

Goldberg, A. (1997). Tailoring to fit: Altering our approach to multicultural populations. *ASHA, 39*(2), 22–28.

Hadley, P. A., & Rice, M. L. (1991). Conversational responsiveness of speech- and language-impaired preschoolers. *Journal of Speech and Hearing Research, 34*, 1308–1317.

Hayes, P. A., Norris, J., & Flaitz, J. R. (1998). Comparison of the oral narrative abilities of underachieving and highachieving gifted adolescents: A preliminary investigation. Language, Speech, and Hearing Services in Schools, 29, 179–187.

Horgan, D. (1978). The development of the full passive. *Journal of Child Language, 5*, 65–80.

Johnson, S. S., & Reichle, J. (1993). Designing and implementing interventions to decrease challenging behavior. *Language, Speech, and Hearing Services in Schools, 24*, 225–235.

Labov, W. (1972). *Language in the inner city: Studies in the Black English Vernacular*. Philadelphia: University of Pennsylvania Press.

Larson, V. L., & McKinley, N. L. (1993). Clinical forum: Adolescent language—an introduction. *Language, Speech, and Hearing Services in Schools, 24*, 19–20.

Larson, V. L., McKinley, N. L., & Boley, D. (1993). Service delivery models for adolescents with language disorders. *Language, Speech, and Hearing Services in Schools, 24*, 36–42.

Mack, A. E., & Warr-Leeper, G. A. (1992). Language abilities in boys with chronic behavior disorders. *Language, Speech, and Hearing Services in Schools, 23*, 214–223.

Masterson, J. J., & Perrey, C. D. (1994). A program for training analogical reasoning skills in children with language disorders. *Language, Speech, and Hearing Disorders in Schools, 25*, 268–270.

Masterson, J. J., & Perrey, C. D. (1999). Training analogical reasoning skills in children with language disorders. *American Journal of Speech-Language Pathology, 8*, 53–61.

McLaughlin, S. (1998). *Introduction to language development*. San Diego, CA: Singular.

Newhoff, M., & Leonard, L. (1983). Diagnosis of developmental language disorders. In I. J. Meitus & B. Weinberg (Eds.), *Diagnosis in speech-language pathology* (pp. 71–112). Baltimore, MD: University Park Press.

Nippold, M. A. (1993). Developmental markers in adolescent language: Syntax, semantics, and pragmatics. *Language, Speech, and Hearing Services in Schools, 24*, 21–29.

Olswang, L. B., Rodriguez, B., & Timler, G. (1998). Recommending intervention for toddlers with specific language learning difficulties:

We may not have all the answers, but we know a lot. *American Journal of Speech-Language Pathology, 7*, 23–32.

Oram, J., Fine, J., Okamoto, C., & Tannock, R. (1999). Assessing the language of children with attention deficit hyperactivity disorder. *American Journal of Speech-Language Pathology, 8*, 72–80.

Owens, R. E., Jr. (1984). *Language development. An Introduction.* Columbus, OH: Merrill.

Parnell, M. M., Amerman, J. D., & Harting, R. D. (1986). Responses of language-disordered children to wh-questions. *Language, Speech, and Hearing Services in Schools, 17*, 95–106.

Peters-Johnson, C. (1992). Fast facts: A look at what is happening in education and the professions. *Language, Speech, and Hearing Services in Schools, 23*, 92.

Qualls, C. D., & Harris, J. L. (1999). Effects of familiarity on idiom comprehension in African American and European American fifth graders. *Language, Speech, and Hearing Services in Schools, 30*, 141–151.

Reed, V. A., McLeod, K., & McAllister, L. (1999). Importance of selected communication skills for talking with peers and teachers: Adolescents' opinions. *Language, Speech, and Hearing Services in Schools, 30*, 32–49.

Rhyner, P. M., Kelly, D. J., Brantley, A. L., & Krueger, D. M. (1999). Screening low-income African American children using the BLT-2S and the SPELT-P. *American Journal of Speech-Language Pathology, 8*, 44–52.

Rice, M. L., Sell, M. A., & Hadley, P. A. (1991). Social interactions of speech- and language-impaired children. *Journal of Speech and Hearing Research, 34*, 1299–1307.

Roseberry-McKibbin, C. (1994). Assessment and intervention for children with limited English proficiency and language disorders. *ASHA, 3*(3), 77–88.

Schuele, C. M., & Hadley, P. A. (1999). Potential advantages of introducing specific language impairment to families. *American Journal of Speech-Language Pathology, 8*, 11–22.

Schwabe, A. M., Olswang, L. B., & Kriegsmann, E. (1986). Requests for information: Linguistic, cognitive, pragmatic, and environmental variables. *Language, Speech, and Hearing Services in Schools, 17*, 38–55.

Seidenberg, P. L., & Bernstein, D. K. (1986). The comprehension of similes and metaphors by learning-disabled and nonlearning-disabled children. *Language, Speech, and Hearing Services in Schools, 17*, 219–229.

Simon, C. S. (1979). *Communicative competence: A functional-pragmatic approach to language therapy.* Tucson, AZ: Communication Skill Builders.

Spector, C. C. (1992). Remediating humor comprehension deficits in language-impaired students. *Language, Speech, and Hearing Services in Schools, 23*, 20–27.

Tager-Flusberg, H. (1985). Putting words together: Morphology and syntax in the preschool years. In J. K. Gleason (Ed.), *The development of language* (pp. 139–171). Columbus, OH: Merrill.

Ukrainetz, T. A. (1998). Stickwriting stories: A quick and easy narrative representation strategy. *Language, Speech, and Hearing Services in Schools, 29*, 197–206.

Washington, J. A., & Craig, H. K. (1999). Performances of at-risk, African American preschoolers on the Peabody Picture Vocabulary Test-III. *Language, Speech, and Hearing Services in Schools, 30*, 75–82.

Webster's beginning dictionary. (1980). Springfield, MA: Merriam.

Westby, C. (1999). *Changing views of ADHD: Roles for speech-language pathologists in evaluation and treatment of students.* ASHA Telephone Seminar: March 25, 1999.

Wiig, E. H. (1986). Language disabilities in school-age children and youth. In G. H. Shames & E. H. Wiig (Eds.), *Human communication disorders* (2nd ed.). (pp. 331–383). Columbus, OH: Merrill.

Wiig, E. H., & Semel, E. (1984). *Language assessment and intervention for the learning disabled* (2nd ed.). Columbus, OH: Merrill.

Wilson, C. C., Lanza, J. R., & Barton, J. S. (1988). Developing higher level thinking skills through questioning techniques in the speech and language setting. *Language, Speech, and Hearing Services in Schools, 19*, 428–431.

Work, R. S., Cline, J. A., Ehren, B. J., Keiser, D. L., & Wujek, C. (1993). Adolescent language programs. *Language, Speech, and Hearing Services in Schools, 24*, 43–53.

Chapter 4

Stuttering

The classroom teacher has the opportunity not only to observe but also to help the child who stutters. The teacher is also in a pivotal position to establish a working relationship between the child who stutters and the other children in the classroom, with the speech-language pathologist and with the parents. Furthermore, through the teacher's knowledgeable and caring leadership the atmosphere in which the child must live and learn can become one that optimizes both cognitive and emotional development.

Anything outside the realm of the expected tends to attract the attention of others. And so it is with stuttering. We expect that speech will move along smoothly and without any radical departures from "normal," although we have all observed that in the speech of most people there are pauses and sometimes repetitions. But when pauses, hesitations, words or sounds are prolonged, or some words are blurted out or distorted, the speech draws adverse attention to itself. In some instances these breaks in the fluency of speech also interfere significantly with the intelligibility of the intended message

Some preschoolers and school-age children show speech disruptions that are labeled "stuttering" when really parents and others who apply this label are observing normal nonfluencies. To be sure, some of these youngsters might one day be stutterers. Most will not.

Over the past 40 years, special education programs have matured within the public schools in the United States. Along with their development has come special attention to those with speech, language, and hearing problems. We are fortunate to have both federal and state educational agencies interested in special problems that interfere with the learning of the school child. We are so accustomed to this specialized help that it seems to be taken for granted. However, in many countries throughout the world such services are not available.

In the United States, clinical services for stutterers, both child and adult, are available through various sources including schools, community clinics, university clinics, hospitals, and private practice settings. The development of these sources of help has been influenced by several factors: (1) the recognition by educators of the need for specialized services, (2) the leadership provided by specialists within colleges and universities who have developed clinical and research programs focused on stuttering, (3) the American Speech-Language-Hearing Association, (4) state speech-language and hearing associations, (5) the Stuttering Foundation of America, and (6) the willingness of the departments of special education at state and federal levels to provide funding for both clinical and research programs.

Regardless of the extent to which programs have or have not been implemented to help children and adults who stutter, this speech problem has been observed for centuries. Clinicians, scientists, and others have attempted to understand stuttering and to develop a methodology for dealing with this communication disorder, the behaviors that frequently accompany it, and the perceptions of those who interact with stutterers. One study suggests that the fear, tension, anxiety, and nervousness that often accompany stuttering are so powerful as to be perceptible even when the stutterer is not speaking (Kalinowski, Stuart, & Armson, 1996).

What Is Known about "Normal" Speech and Stuttering?

There has been a great deal of discussion and study among clinicians and researchers involved with stuttering on the topics of fluent speech, nonfluent speech, and stuttering. Although these topics have been the subjects of numerous investigations, not all of the answers are obvious at this time, although good progress is being made.

What Is Fluent Speech?

Speech that moves along easily and without undue interruptions is thought by most of us to be fluent speech. Perhaps the reader is aware of people who really are not all that fluent but who are not stutterers.

It has been thought by some that fluency was somehow associated with linguistic proficiency, that is, the ability to select the proper word, to pronounce words correctly, to arrange them in correct sequence within the sentence, or to use a word that is appropriate to the situation. All of these factors might indeed bear upon fluency, but it must be realized as well that people who stutter and those who do not might have similar problems. Thus, the classroom teacher, parent, or anyone else who interacts with the child whose speech is nonfluent must be cautious about attributing the lack of fluency to inadequate handling of the language.

Probably all of us, depending upon the situation, are sometimes less fluent than at other times. Surprise, shock, excitement, disbelief, and other emotions can all contribute momentarily to some deterioration in fluency. It would be the rare individual who never manifested anything but smooth speech devoid of any repetitions, pauses, or hesitations. Momentary lapses in fluency are, however, exceptional and infrequent occurrences in the speech of the normal speaker.

So, in answer to the question "What is fluent speech?," it is speech that is:

- Relatively effortless
- Not punctuated with many irregularities such as repetitions, hesitations, or prolongations
- Relatively free of abnormal pauses or discontinuities
- Rhythmic and easy as it moves forward

What Is Stuttering?

One day there might be agreement on the answer to this question, but for the present there is still much to be learned. It is not because clinicians and researchers have not addressed this question, for a tremendous amount of clinical observation, description of stuttering behavior, and empirical research has been carried on for years. As one would expect, these efforts have yielded some excellent insights that have provided the bases for many fine therapy programs structured for children and also adults.

To define anything implies that what the definition says about the defined substance, process, concept, or whatever is all that there is to be said. Thus, right now it is best to view definitions of stuttering as operational definitions only, which provide points of reference against which to attempt to explain causation and a substrate upon which to develop programs of intervention.

Some would attempt to shed more definitive light on stuttering by noting the behavioral symptoms that accompany stuttering. Prolongations and repetitions of sounds, syllables, and words or abnormally long pauses are some of these behaviors. Avoidance of sounds, words, and situations and increased anxiety are also part of the picture. Those who work in research or clinical programs are quite aware of the behaviors that accompany stuttering. It should be noted as well that many who are not trained listeners can also detect stuttering when it occurs. The classroom teacher who is with children many hours each day is in a particularly advantageous position to identify and refer those who stutter to the speech-language pathologist.

Identifying normal disfluencies and abnormal disfluencies presents a challenge to the listener who would attempt to differentiate the stuttering child from the nonstutterer. The observation of struggle behavior has been one of the criteria for doing so. A recent study (Armson et al., 1997) found good agreement between the ratings of listeners who listened to disfluent speech of children and rated them as fluent or disfluent and other listeners who rated them on a 7-point scale relative to their fluency. The researchers suggest that "as the perception of degree of *struggle* increased, so did the likelihood that the disfluent production would be judged as stuttered" (p.42).

The number of repetitions of sounds, syllables, words, or phrases that occur in a child's speech has also been used to differentiate stuttering from normal nonfluency. A recent study (Ambrose & Yairi, 1995) that derived data from 29 children in each of two groups (experimental and control) speaking approximately 28,000 syllables confirms the idea that the number of repetitions does indeed assist in the differentiation of stuttering children from normally nonfluent children. It should be noted, however, that repetitions are only one parameter by which one identifies stuttering from normal disfluency, albeit an important one.

As suggested earlier, there is still much to be learned about stuttering despite years of observations made by clinicians and research scientists. Various theories have developed over the years. A logical question is what will research in stuttering and clinical observations yield in the years to come. For example, Perkins (1994) notes that the matter of "loss of control" of speech by the stutterer has not been included in current theories. This and other areas will undoubtedly receive close attention in the twenty-first century. In addition to the studies made by scientists in the laboratory setting, anecdotal observations made by clinicians and teachers will also spur advances. The classroom teacher can help advance the body of knowledge about stuttering by maintaining a close relationship with the speech-language pathologist while teaching a child within the classroom who stutters.

What Causes Stuttering?

Even though the historical interest in stuttering dates back several centuries, the search continues for the causes of this challenging speech disorder. Scientists and clinicians have looked seriously at this problem and the results of their observations and experimentation can be found in the literature both in the United States and abroad. Hypotheses and theories of causation stem from this effort. To describe *how* stuttering occurs is one thing; however, to ascertain the factors that cause it to occur is quite another. Nonetheless, the descriptions of stuttering can be useful in designing programs to help the stutterer modify certain behaviors.

Historical Perspectives

One interesting approach to the question of causation of stuttering was offered over 50 years ago by Johnson (1948), who suggested that stuttering was in the ear of the listener. That is to say, when one labels the disfluencies of a child as stuttering, the one who labels and those who surround the child respond to the child as though stuttering is occurring. Eventually the child also responds to the disfluencies as stuttering. It should be noted that this theory of causation may have something to recommend it, but most scientists and clinicians are examining other possible causative factors.

For many years, Van Riper (1972), a prominent leader in the field of stuttering and a highly successful clinician, suggested that stuttering had many origins and that the factors that *maintain* the stuttering are more important than those thought to be the original causes. This rather eclectic orientation formed the substrate of his theoretical framework and approach to therapy.

A different point of view, held by Perkins (1986), is that stuttering results from the discoordination of respiration, voicing, and articulation. He maintained that the discoordination interfered with the precision of time of air flow and vocalization. This, he states, is not the cause of stuttering but *is* the stuttering; the cause is some underlying constitutional condition.

Gregory (1986) in his comprehensive review of disfluency and stuttering presented findings from areas important to stuttering. These include family history, auditory processing, speech motor processes, language factors, environmental factors, and electroencephalography.

In his analytical review of theoretical approaches to causation of stuttering, Ham (1990) categorized the general themes under which theories of stuttering have emerged through the years. Three categories emerged from his analysis: psychological, linguistic, and pathophysiological.

The *psychological* category included psychoanalytic considerations wherein the stuttering is perceived as a symptom of some underlying neurosis and also psychosocial considerations (such as those spoken of by Johnson, 1948) wherein stuttering tends to increase if rewarded and to decrease if the stuttering elicits punishment. Of all the approaches that are psychologically based, the learned behavior approach has received the greatest attention from clinicians and researchers.

Of interest within the psychological category are recent findings that adult stutterers report a significantly higher number of daily stressors than control groups of nonstutterers (Blood et al., 1997). These findings are consistent with data from another study in which the subjects who were stutterers showed a proportional increment in stuttering as a result of stress induced artificially in the laboratory (Caruso et al., 1994).

A recent study highlights the psychological effects of speech-associated attitudes of children who stutter as contrasted with children who do not stutter (Vanryckeghem & Brutten, 1997). Fifty-five children who stuttered and 55 who did not were administered the Communication Attitude Test (C.A.T.), a true-false test that sampled their attitudes toward their own speech. There were noticeable differences between those who stuttered and those who did not. Those who stuttered had poorer attitudes toward their speech experiences than those who did not stutter. Furthermore, these poor attitudes tended to increase with age.

Considerations related to *linguistics* as a causative factor have led to evaluation of the role of language development as it affects stuttering. The complexity of syntax, frequency and predictability of words, linguistic stress, phonology, and semantics are all important variables in the relationship of a child's language development to stuttering. For example, one study demonstrated that there are more articulation/phonological problems among children who stutter than among normally fluent children matched by age and sex (Paden & Yairi, 1996).

Language is most dominant in the left hemisphere of the brain in most people; therefore, *pathophysiological* considerations are not to be overlooked. Many studies have been made over the past seven decades attempting to relate stuttering to some neurophysiological base. Some have contended that stutterers have a tendency toward equality of cerebral dominance. This implies that when speech is attempted, the coordination of the hemispheres is affected, causing a disruption of the control of the speech mechanism. The advent of more sophisticated testing devices such as magnetoencephalography and magnetic resonance imaging (MRI) and more knowledge of the functioning of the brain as related to cortical activation has enhanced investigations into the role of cerebral dominance.

A neurophysiological study (Morgan, Cranford, & Burk, 1997) that focused on stutterers versus nonstutterers attempted to determine whether or not there was a difference between the two groups in relation to the P300 event-related potential, which reflects cognitive functioning. The investigators found that some of the stutterers showed different patterns of interhemispheric activity than did the nonstutterers. They suggest that this finding lends support to the possibility of altered cerebral dominance in some forms of stuttering.

It has been noted for many years that stuttering seems to run in families (Yairi, Ambrose, & Cox, 1996). Thus, as with studies of cerebral dominance, there is also a rather extensive literature providing some evidence that there is a *genetic component* related to stuttering. Why some stutterers seem to overcome or recover from their stuttering early in childhood and why others persist in their stuttering is a question that has generated great interest.

There is a difference in the *gender* of those who recover and those who do not. Females are less apt to continue stuttering than are their male counterparts. This statement is borne out by the results of one study (Ambrose, Cox, & Yairi, 1997) that indicates a dramatic difference in sex ratios of persistent versus recovered stutterers; recovery is more frequent among the females than among males. They also found that recovery or persistence in stuttering is transmitted genetically and also that recovery is not a milder form of stuttering. However, that which is seen as milder stuttering and the more persistent stuttering are not independent genetically; both stem from a common genetic cause, and the persistence is partially due to additional genetic factors.

Although genetic factors are very important in the search for causes of stuttering, environmental factors should not be ignored. Psychosocial influences in the home, school, and other settings are important and should be taken into consideration as analyses are made of those factors that might cause an otherwise normally nonfluent child to persist in nonfluent speech patterns.

Respiration of stutterers has been another area of inquiry. It appears that irregularities in respiration are associated with stuttering rather than being a causative factor.

Upon review of the various areas of inquiry (psychological, linguistic, and pathophysiological), one sees clearly that stuttering is etiologically multifaceted. As research continues, one can expect that there will be more definitive information derived in all of the areas and that there will be a better understanding as to the relationships among them.

Do Cultural Factors Influence Stuttering?

The United States is considered to be an ethnic melting pot, rich in a variety of cultural patterns, religious beliefs, and political perspectives. This kind of diversity gives us a splendid opportunity to compare our particular orientations with those of others about us. One of the things we observe is that some of our neighbors have long since lost track of exactly where their roots lie. Others, however, cling tenaciously to their countries and languages of origin and preserve their native cultures by living in close proximity to others of the same origin. Habits, traditions, attitudes, and ultimately the values they have inherited become fixed, despite the New World setting in which they find themselves. These then are handed down from generation to generation (Perspectives, 1990).

Recognizing the impact of cultural influences on the rehabilitation of communication disorders and sensing the need for more dialogue on this topic, various publications, for example, by Screen and Anderson (1994) and Kayser (1998), have been developed to draw specific attention to the importance of understanding multiculturalism as related to assessment and intervention. It is important to note that attitudes influenced by cultural backgrounds can have a profound influence on how parents and others in the family and immediate surroundings react to a child who stutters. Likewise, they can have an important influence on how parents and others respond to the suggestions they receive from those who are trying to help the child.

This presents a unique challenge to both the classroom teacher and the speech-language pathologist. This brings to mind an experience that the writer once had with a father (within a particular ethnic group) of a son who stuttered. The father was invited to come to the school with his wife and other parents to discuss the progress that their children were making in speech therapy. He was convinced that his son needed no help and articulated his feelings about it quite vigorously. It was obvious that his sense of pride and also ignorance of his son's need motivated his behavior. Wanting to help him and at the same time wanting to continue to provide therapy to his son, I took great care to explain to him the needs of his son and what was being done in therapy for his child. Fortunately he had an understanding wife who seemed to be quite accepting of therapy for her son. Her help and the effort made to communicate with the father happily resulted in his becoming a very supportive individual in the therapy process.

As a classroom teacher in a diverse society, it is important to be sensitive to cultural differences. Perhaps you have children in your classroom who come from homes that have cultural values that set them apart from the majority of the other children, and it might be that some of those children need special attention because of stuttering. Before making judgments as to the next steps for the child who stutters, make an appraisal along with the speech-language pathologist of the cultural background of the child. Do not engage in stereotyping; always be aware that there are subcultures within cultural groups and that there are individual differences among children.

Is There Help for the Child Who Stutters?

Clinical observations and research studies both indicate that the answer to this question is yes. However, it is useful to think of two general age categories as we examine the possibility of treatment. One category is the preschool child and the other is the child of school age. The teacher at both levels has a role to play with children showing disfluencies. The important thing to determine at the outset is when and when not to intervene with a program focused on the speech behavior of the child. The speech-language pathologist formulates decisions about the need for intervention while interviewing the child. Among the instruments that have been constructed to facilitate this process, for example, are those by Riley (1998) on predicting stuttering and Thompson (1998) on the assessment of fluency.

Curlee and Yairi (1997) cite incidence figures for stuttering in the United States and western Europe to be approximately 4 percent to 5 percent and the prevalence figures at about 0.5 percent to 1.0 percent. Their data show that those children who stopped stuttering are generally younger when they begin, have fewer relatives who stutter, and are girls. Curlee (1991) has suggested that most people who are ever going to stutter will begin stuttering before their fifth birthday and that virtually no one begins stuttering after age 12 unless there has been serious head trauma.

How does one differentiate the young child who stutters from the child with nonfluent speech who will recover? Research data (Curlee & Yairi, 1998) indicate that when there is uncertainty as to whether or not a child stutters, a systematic period of assessment of the child's speech should be undertaken. This is not always an easy task, but there are some important cues to observe. If the child with nonfluent speech talks easily and does not seem to be bothered by it or show struggle behavior, the likelihood is that one is viewing a child who will cease stuttering. The results of credible studies indicate that *most* children who begin to stutter will stop without receiving treatment (Curlee & Yairi, 1997). Some will continue to stutter for as long as 2 or more years after the onset. It is these children who are at risk for stuttering as adults. It is largely held that the longer a child has been stuttering, the greater the likelihood that the child will not recover unless some specialized help is provided (Zebrowski, 1997). A waiting period (when the clinician is not sure whether to place the stuttering child in trial therapy, hoping for spontaneous recovery) is a perfect period for clinician, teacher, and parents to gather additional data that could be useful in determining whether stuttering is increasing or decreasing for a particular child (Ingham & Cordes, 1998).

An interesting question arises as to whether or not the speech of those who recover without formal help in a program is perceived as being no different from those who never stuttered. Research indicates that children who recover without any formal treatment have speech that is no different perceptually from that of the children who never showed signs of stuttering or serious disfluency (Finn et al., 1997).

The reports of parents are important. Parents who are concerned with the disfluency of a child should be made aware that they can definitely be of help by focusing their attention on what the child is saying, not how the child is saying it. However, if parents report that the speech behavior of their child is characterized by frequent repetitions and prolongations and that there is considerable struggle involved, then the child should definitely be referred to the speech-language pathologist for further observation and possible treatment. The attitudes of parents are very important also. If they add to the discomfort being expressed by the child through obvious signs of nonacceptance of the child's speech, this only exacerbates the situation for the child. The clinician will want to deal with this in the evaluative process. No longer do professionals tiptoe around the stuttering of a child for fear of calling attention to the problem. Two things should be remembered: (1) If the child is experiencing stuttering as a problem, there is indeed already an awareness of it; and (2) the sooner a child receives help for stuttering, the better, for it has been shown that early treatment yields the best results (Perkins, 1991).

Some have advocated the use of a trial period of therapy for more indepth observation of the disfluencies in the speech of the preschool child, and also as a way to decrease those disfluencies. It is important to determine just what should occur in the trial therapy period and to be able to describe what has been accomplished.

The approaches employed in the management of the school-age stutterer are similar to those employed with the preschooler. However, the age range for the school-age child is of course greater than that of the preschooler. Those in the lower end of the primary grades are much more similar to the preschooler, whereas at the upper end of the school-age range the similarity is more like that of the adolescent or adult. One can well imagine the many different approaches that are employed with hundreds of stuttering children across the country and world-wide. A few examples include the *operant treatment approach*, which includes the use of "prolonged speech" to give the stuttering child a novel speech pattern that is subsequently shaped toward more natural-sounding speech; and the *stutter more fluently* approach, which attempts to help the child cope more effectively with the stuttering rather than attempting to eliminate it (Lincoln, Onslow, & Reed, 1996). Another approach utilizes a *response-contingent time-out* strategy that demands a 5-second pause when stuttering occurs. This approach shows promise (Onslow et al., 1997). An interesting comparison of several methods is reported by clinicians in Australia who used *intensive smooth speech, electromyography feedback,* and *home-based smooth speech.* All three methods were reported as being "very successful" (Craig et al., 1996).

Of course, an important criterion to be used in judging whether a method has been successful is the extent to which sophisticated (clinicians) and unsophisticated listeners can tell the difference in the speech of children who have never stuttered and those who have undergone treatment and have recovered. This is a *social validity* criterion. Several researchers have put this notion to the test under well-controlled conditions and have shown rather conclusively that the employment of a particular method (an operant treatment program called the Lidcombe Program) they employed was indeed successful with the children (Lincoln et al., 1997). Still another criterion is that of *communicative suitability* of speech. Researchers in The Netherlands developed and evaluated a test instrument for just this purpose. Ten different communication situations were used in their study. Their findings suggest that their instrument provides reliable results and that communicative suitability is a promising criterion to investigate further (Franken, Van Bezooijen, & Boves, 1997).

An outstanding need is for documentation of treatment effectiveness so that best approaches can be shared. Guidelines for such documentation have been suggested (Ingham & Riley, 1998) that could be applicable to any treatment and would be helpful in verifying effects of treatment.

Interacting with the nonfluent or stuttering child of school age usually comes before the clinician has had an opportunity to hold an interview with the parents. This makes for a different starting point when talking with the parents for the first time. It must be emphasized that success with therapy for children within this age range necessitates bringing the parents into the picture and allowing them to express their concerns. Of importance as well is giving parents a chance to share their attitudes toward the child and the child's speech behavior.

In order to determine what steps should be taken, it is necessary to make an evaluation of the speech of the stuttering or nonfluent child and perhaps set up a trial period of therapy. This provides the opportunity to address both the matter of fluency and the stuttering behavior. Properly handled, the child can be made aware of the problem of fluency and stuttering objectively and can thus be desensitized, decreasing or diminishing the fears, anxieties, and stigma associated with the stuttering.

Does the classroom teacher have a role to play here? Indeed so! The teacher plays a vital role in the lives of all children in the classroom and particularly in the lives of those who exhibit nonfluent speech or who stutter. These children are vulnerable. They are vulnerable to the misconceptions, attitudes, and responses of others, both children and adults. When there is proper management and understanding promoted within the classroom by the teacher tremendous progress can be made. The teacher has great control over the psychosocial environment of the classroom and can counter negative reactions from the children toward the child who stutters. When negative attitudes surface, the teacher has a window of opportunity to explain to the classmates that when the disfluent child has some difficulty talking, they can be of real help to him or her by listening carefully. Even though children can be very cruel to each other, they can also be very cooperative and accepting if the right leadership is provided that elicits their support.

It is well to note the perspective of Perkins (1991), who suggests that if stuttering persists into adulthood, both professionals and those who stutter may look only to improvements in their stuttering. Their speech might sound normal most of the time, but they might still perceive themselves as stutterers. Thus, if help can be provided to children *before* they begin to fear stuttering and before they develop other kinds of secondary reactions such as blinking, facial grimaces, et cetera, the chances are good that they will become reasonably normal speakers. Preventing a self-image of being a stutterer is of great importance. The classroom teacher can assist significantly in this process.

Case Histories

Sammy

Sammy was a rather shy fifth-grader who was new in the elementary school. He had a moderate stuttering problem that his classroom teacher noted on the first day he appeared. He transferred into the school in December from a school in a rather remote area of the state. He had been enrolled there since the first grade.

Immediately upon noticing the difficulty he was having with speaking, the classroom teacher contacted the speech-language pathologist, who contacted the parents and after an evaluation, suggested that Sammy be enrolled for therapy. He received individual therapy once a week and group therapy twice each week. The classroom teacher gave him excellent support within the classroom. There were two other students in his classroom who were also receiving special help for their speech problems, so the other children were aware of speech problems, which was helpful to Sammy. Sammy made excellent progress with his stuttering problem through the expert guidance of the speech-language pathologist, who worked closely with the classroom teacher. By the end of the school year in May his speech was much improved and his adjustment to the activities of the classroom excellent.

Jack

Jack was in the second grade and doing very well in school. Both of his parents were active professional people, and he had no brothers or sisters. About 5 months into the school year Jack developed a rapid-fire, machine-gun–like stuttering over the course of 2 weeks. He had blocks, repetitions, and facial grimaces. His father (a speech-language-pathologist) was concerned because in Jack's bedtime prayers, Jack prayed that he would be able to complete his work the next day in school. It was also noted that Jack had been watching many hours of television each day. At a parent–teacher conference, Jack's father and teacher discussed Jack's progress in school and the hope expressed in Jack's prayers. When asked about Jack's ability to complete his work, the teacher (young and inexperienced) said, "Oh yes, he completes his work far ahead of the rest of the students, so I simply enrich his activities with more work than he can complete." Because of the "enrichment," Jack was never able to go to the sand table and play with others who had completed their routine assignments. At the father's request, Jack's assignments were reduced to normal and Jack was rewarded by being able to play at the sand table upon their completion.

Additionally, Jack and his parents decided together the television programs he would watch and for how long. The parents curtailed some of their own activities and spent more time with Jack individually in play activities. It was not more than 3 weeks before the "stuttering" subsided and was never observed again. Sensitive parents, a good analysis of the probable causative factors, and a cooperative classroom teacher played vital roles in the restoration of fluency in this youngster. The situation might have been quite different if prompt action had not been taken.

Susie

Susie was an easy, relaxed stutterer. Before speech-language pathologists were available in all schools, her fourth-grade teacher decided that Susie should talk more fluently and set about to correct her speech by having her stop and start over each time she repeated a syllable or word. Additionally, the teacher appointed "watchdogs" from among the students to "assist" her not only in the classroom but also on the playground. Susie was miserable. At age 18 and ready to graduate from high school, she was a well-entrenched stutterer with all the frustrations, fears, and anxieties that might have been avoided had there been a speech-language pathologist in the school who could have worked with Susie and her parents in close cooperation with the classroom teacher.

David

David was a delightful 4-year-old preschooler. His father, a surgeon, and his mother, a psychologist, brought the child to the clinic for evaluation of his "stuttering." The father insisted that the child needed evaluation and was quite concerned about the status of his only son, who was developing normally in all respects except for his speech. This had been confirmed by a neurological examination at the Speech and Hearing Clinic. The father was "high-strung" and perfectionistic. This was the unspoken observation of the speech-language pathologist, which the mother reinforced indirectly several times during the interview. The mother appeared calm and relaxed and not overly concerned about David's speech disfluencies and suggested that they might be a part of the normal development picture.

David was seen briefly in a play situation both with and without the parents being present. He was showing easy disfluencies in speech that were not accompanied by any sense of fear of speaking or struggle in the production of words or sentences. He interacted well with the speech-language pathologist and appeared to be at ease and happy.

In the first of three interviews held over the course of 3 months with the parents it was suggested to them that what they were noting were normal disfluencies and that they should refrain from reacting to them as stuttering. It was further suggested, however, that they continue to observe David's speech and note when the disfluencies were most apparent. Additionally it was suggested that if there were pressures on David that could be alleviated, the needed adjustments should be made. They were counseled as well to spend more time with David; listen closely to what he said to them; and to become engaged meaningfully with him in play, reading of stories, et cetera.

By the third interview both parents seemed pleased with the suggestions made and reported that they thought they noticed much greater fluency in David's speech. Also it became apparent to the clinician that the father had really begun to enjoy his preschool son as a person. The speech-language pathologist and the parents agreed during the third interview that further interviews were not necessary unless they felt the need for them.

About 3 months after the last interview, around Christmas time, the florist delivered a large poinsettia plant to the home of the speech-language pathologist with a note from the parents expressing their gratitude for helping David along the way to fluent speech. (What was said by the speech-language pathologist over the course of three interviews was essentially what was said in the first interview. It was noted, however, that there was a reluctance on the part of the father to accept the fact that the child's speech was probably characterized by normal disfluency and not "stuttering." By the end of the last interview it was quite apparent that there was acceptance.)

Summary

Some Important Points to Remember

- Current thinking suggests that stuttering has multiple causes.
- Many theories of causation of stuttering exist.
- Three areas of inquiry command the attention of scientists who seek causes of stuttering: psychological, linguistic, and pathophysiological.
- There are important differences between normal speech disfluency and stuttering.
- It is important to differentiate normal disfluency from stuttering.
- Discoordination of respiration, voicing, and articulation are frequently associated with stuttering.
- Early intervention with stuttering children is recommended.
- Most stuttering begins with easy syllable repetitions.
- Facial grimaces and struggle behaviors sometimes accompany stuttering, as do fear, frustration, and hostility.
- Disfluency is often overcome.
- It is important to know which children will probably outgrow nonfluent speech.
- More boys than girls stutter.
- Children who stutter do not all respond alike to the stress connected with stuttering.
- Stuttering interferes with the forward flow of speech.
- Children often stutter more in some situations than in others.
- Some children who stutter feel quite anxious.
- Children with speech disfluencies or stuttering should not be stopped and told to start over or complimented for fluent speech.
- There is some evidence of a genetic component related to stuttering.
- The search continues relative to cerebral dominance and stuttering.
- Various methods have been developed to assist in therapy with the stutterer.
- Parents play a key role in therapy with stuttering children.
- The classroom teacher is very important in dealing with stuttering children.

"Do"s and "Don't"s for Teachers

"Do"s

- Accept the child who stutters just as you would any other child.
- If you observe that a child has marked disfluencies, contact the speech-language pathologist serving your school. Describe your observation of the child's speech and provide all of the pertinent information that is requested.
- Following the evaluation by the speech-language pathologist, find out how you can assist the child in your classroom.
- Try to help build the self-confidence of the child.
- Provide ample opportunity for the child who stutters to participate successfully in oral activities.

- Monitor periodically the free play of the child who stutters to determine the level of peer acceptance and to detect any overt behavior by others that might be associated with the speech problem.
- Maintain eye contact when a child who stutters speaks; be a good listener, even though it may take longer.
- If appropriate, take the opportunity to educate classmates of the child who stutters about stuttering and to help them develop accepting attitudes.
- Reward a child who stutters for things done well, just as you reward any other child.
- Hold the standards high for good manners in talking in the classroom as in other areas of social interactions.
- Stuttering affords no reason why a child should not abide by all of the rules set for other children in the classroom.
- Provide the child who stutters the opportunity to say what he or she has to say.

"Don't"s

- Do not speak for the child when stuttering occurs.
- Do not compliment a child for fluent speech.
- Do not allow interruptions of a child's attempt to speak.
- Do not allow other children to try to furnish a word or sentence that the child who stutters is trying to say.
- Do not ask the child to slow down, stop, or start over.
- Do not give the child who stutters special privileges, with the exception of special assistance in oral recitation when needed.

Referral Sources

- Speech-language pathologist
- Audiologist
- Psychologist

Self-Test

True or False

1. The speech of normal talkers shows no disfluencies.   _____

2. There are multiple causes of stuttering.   _____

3. There are numerous theories of stuttering.   _____

4. More girls stutter than boys.   _____

5. Easy repetitions most frequently characterize the beginning of stuttering in children.   _____

6. Some stutterers regain fluent speech.   _____

7. After identifying a child who seems to be stuttering, the classroom teacher should contact the speech-language pathologist. _____

8. Building self-esteem in a child who stutters is a responsibility of the classroom teacher. _____

9. Stuttering is a serious speech disorder that should receive immediate attention. _____

10. When a child blocks on a sound or a word, the classroom teacher should speak for the child. _____

11. Research in stuttering continues. _____

12. The classroom teacher should praise a stutterer for fluent speech. _____

13. The classroom teacher should help to develop positive attitudes of others toward the child who stutters. _____

14. Only in recent years has stuttering been noticed as a speech problem. _____

15. Cultural diversity should be of concern to teachers. _____

16. Linguistic disfluency and stuttering may be related. _____

17. Only highly trained listeners can detect disfluent speech. _____

18. Some say there might be an inherited predisposition to stuttering. _____

19. Teachers should be sensitive to the cultural backgrounds of children who stutter. _____

20. Children with speech disfluencies should be encouraged to participate in oral recitations. _____

References

Ambrose, N., Cox, N., & Yairi, E. (1997). The genetic basis of persistence and recovery in stuttering. *Journal of Speech, Language, and Hearing Research, 40,* 567–580.

Ambrose, N., & Yairi, E. (1995). The role of repetition units in the differential diagnosis of early childhood incipient stuttering. *Journal of Speech-Language Pathology, 4,* 82–88.

Armson, J., Jenson, S., Gallant, D., Kalinowski, J., & Fee, E. (1997). The relationship between degree of audible struggle and judgments of childhood disfluencies as stuttered or not stuttered. *American Journal of Speech-Language Pathology, 6,* 42–50.

Blood, H., Wertz, H., Blood G., Bennet, S., & Simpson, K. (1997). The effects of life stressors and daily stressors on stuttering. *Journal of Speech, Language, and Hearing Research, 4,* 134–143.

Caruso, A., Chodzkozajko, W., Bidinger, & Sommers, R. (1994). Adults who stutter: Responses to cognitive stress. *Journal of Speech and Hearing Research, 37,* 746–754.

Craig, A., Hancock, K., Chang, E., McReady, C., Shepley, A., McCaul, A., Costello, D., Harding, S., Kehren, R., Masel, C., & Reilly, K. (1996). A controlled clinical trial for stuttering in persons aged 9 to 14 years. *Journal of Speech and Hearing Research, 39,* 808–826.

Curlee, F. (1991). Does my child stutter? In *Stuttering and your child: Questions and answers,* (ch. 9). Memphis, TN: Stuttering Foundation of America.

Curlee, F., & Yairi, E. (1997). Early intervention with early childhood stuttering: A critical examination of the data. *American Journal of Speech-Language Pathology, 6*, 8–18.

Curlee, F., & Yairi, E. (1998). Treatment of early childhood stuttering: Advances and research needs. *Journal of Speech-Language Pathology, 7*, 20–26.

Finn, P., Ingham, R., Ambrose, N., & Yairi, E. (1997). Children recovered from stuttering without formal treatment: Perceptual assessment of speech normalcy. *Journal of Speech, Language, and Hearing Research, 40*, 867–876.

Franken, M., van Bezooijen, R., & Boves, L. (1997). Stuttering and suitability of speech. *Journal of Speech, Language, and Hearing Research, 40*, 83.

Gregory, H. (1986). Stuttering: An integration of contemporary therapies. *Folia Phoniatrica, 38*, 89–120.

Ham, R. (1990). *Therapy of Stuttering*. Englewood Cliffs, NJ: Prentice-Hall.

Ingham, R., & Cordes, A. K. (1998). Treatment decisions for young children who stutter: Further concerns and complexities. *American Journal of Speech Language Pathology, 7*, 15.

Ingham, R., & Riley, G. (1998). Guidelines for documentation of treatment efficacy for young children who stutter. *Journal of Speech, Language, and Hearing Research, 41*, 753.

Johnson, W. (Ed). (1948). *Speech Handicapped School Children*. New York: Harper, 1948.

Kalinowski, J., Stuart, A., & Armson, J. (1996). Perceptions of stutterers and nonstutterers during speaking and nonspeaking situations. *American Journal of Speech-Language Pathology, 5*, (2), 61–67.

Kayser, H. (1998). *Assessment and intervention resource for Hispanic children*. San Diego, CA: Singular Publishing Group.

Lincoln, M., Onslow, M., Lewis, C., & Wilson, L. (1996). A clinical trial of an operant treatment for school-age children who stutter. *American Journal of Speech-Language Pathology, 5*, 73.

Lincoln, M., Onslow, M., & Reed, V. (1997). Social validity of the treatment outcomes of an early intervention program for stuttering. *American Journal of Speech-Language Pathology, 6*, 77.

Morgan, M., Cranford, J., & Burk, K. (1997). P300 event-related potentials in stutterers and non-

stutterers. *Journal of Speech, Language, and Hearing Research, 40*, 1334–1340.

Onslow, M., Packman, A., Stocker, S., van Doorn, J., & Siegel, G. (1997). Control of children's stuttering with response-contingent time-out: Behavioral, perceptual, and acoustic data. *Journal of Speech, Language, and Hearing Research, 40*, 121–133.

Paden, E., & Yairi, E. (1996). Phonological characteristics of children whose stuttering persisted or recovered. *Journal of Speech and Hearing Research, 39*, 981–990.

Perkins, W. (1986). Discoordination of phonation with articulation and respiration. In G. H. Shames & H. Rubin, *Stuttering then and now* (Ch. 4, postscript). Columbus, OH: Merrill.

Perkins, W. (1991). Should we seek help? In *Stuttering and your child: Questions and answers* (Ch. 7). Memphis, TN: Stuttering Foundation of America.

Perkins, W. (1994). Solving unsolvable stuttering. *American Journal of Speech-Language Pathology, 3*, 32–33.

Perspectives. (1990). *The ASHA Office of Minority Concerns Newsletter, 11*, 4. Rockville, MD: American Speech, Language and Hearing Association.

Riley, G. (1998). Stuttering prediction instrument for young children. *Pro-Ed*, Fall Catalog.

Screen, R., & Anderson, N. (1994). *Multicultural perspectives in communication disorders*. San Diego, CA: Singular Publishing Group.

Thompson, J. (1998). Assessment of fluency in school-age children. *Pro-Ed*, Fall Catalog.

Van Riper, C. (1972). *Speech correction principles and methods*. Englewood Cliffs, NJ: Prentice-Hall.

Vanryckeghem, M., & Brutten, G. (1997). The speech-associated attitude of children who do and do not stutter and the differential effect of age. *American Journal of Speech-Language Pathology, 6*, 67–73.

Yairi, E., Ambrose, N., & Cox, N. (1996). Genetics of stuttering: A critical review. *Journal of Speech and Hearing Research, 39*, 771–784.

Zebrowski, P. (1997). Assisting young children who stutter and their families: Defining the role of the speech-language pathologist. *American Journal of Speech-Language Pathology, 6*, 23.

Chapter 5

Voice Disorders

Each one of us has a voice that is unique. It is in some measure a reflection of our personalities. It is unique in that it varies from person to person not only in relation to our personalities but also in relation to our individual and rather complex voice-producing mechanisms. How often have you answered the phone and immediately have been able to identify the caller, just from the voice? Or think of the times that you have listened to the radio or television and have identified the talkers, not from a visual image, but from their voices alone.

One's voice also frequently reflects one's current emotional state. Elation, sadness, fear, anxiety, disbelief, and anger can be obvious to the listener. Of course, you can modify your voice to suit a specific occasion. Perhaps you simply want to portray a voice of another person—not hard to do if you try. Actors and actresses become masters of this as they are called upon to portray various characters.

The voice we produce is "overlaid" on an anatomical structure, the basic function of which is to protect the airway to the lungs and assist in some other important functions.

Some voices are pleasant and others are quite unpleasant. Some talkers sound as though they are talking through their nose—very nasal. Others sound as though they constantly have a head cold, for example " dow we bust go hob" for "now we must go home"—very denasal. Some have pitches that are too high and some too low. Some voices are harsh, and others hoarse. Any of these types of voice problems can distract the listener from what is actually being said.

Some voice problems are associated with medical or general health conditions. Some vocal habits that result in unpleasant voices are learned. An individual's social acceptance and credibility can be greatly influenced by the pleasantness or unpleasantness of the voice.

Do Many Children Have Voice Disorders?

Estimates of voice disorders among children vary substantially by as much as approximately 22 percent. Wilson (1987) has stated that most incidence surveys have found that 6 percent–9 percent of all children have voice disorders. Therefore, out of a class of 30 children there would be 1 or 2 children who would exhibit a voice disorder. Is there a gender difference? Yes, boys are more likely to have voice disorders than girls, and the majority of them occur in the primary grades.

Voice cases are not proportionally represented on caseloads of speech-language pathologists. Why not? Some have speculated that parents and teachers grow accustomed to the unusual voice of a child and tend to associate it with the child and do not think of it as a voice disorder—that's just the way Susie talks! Therefore, speech-language pathologists in the schools who rely on teacher referrals do not receive the referrals; thus, their caseloads reflect fewer voice cases than might be expected.

Sometimes parents and teachers miss identifying a voice problem because they are aware that allergies, colds, or sore throats can cause the voice to sound less than pleasant. These conditions are normally temporary and are expected to pass. Thus, no serious attention is paid to them, and the child unfortunately goes unnoticed, undocumented, and untreated.

Occasionally classroom teachers have available to them inservice education programs that focus on speech and voice problems. It is highly recommended that teachers participate in these programs as a part of their continuing education. They can help the teacher to become more sensitive to voice problems of children and to make well-informed referrals to the speech-language pathologist.

When Should a Child Be Referred to a Speech-Language Pathologist?

A classroom teacher should feel free to refer a child to the speech-language pathologist if there is *any doubt* in his or her mind whether the child has a voice problem. Perhaps the child's voice is hoarse or husky or perhaps the pitch of the voice seems too low or too high for the child's age and gender. If the quality of the child's voice sounds unpleasant or the volume does not seem appropriate, the classroom teacher should seek the advice of the speech-language pathologist. The teacher is in a strategic position to get help for the child and to ask for professional appraisal and advice.

Are There Different Kinds of Voice Disorders?

Yes, there are several kinds of voice disorders that can be observed among children. To describe all of them fully would go considerably beyond the scope of this chapter. Therefore, only the most prominent will be discussed.

Voice disorders are associated with the basic processes that operate to produce voice and are observed in the dimensions of pitch, loudness, and quality. It is within this frame of reference that the following problems are reviewed.

When can one say that a voice disorder exists? A voice disorder exists when a speaker's voice differs significantly from "normal" in pitch, in loudness, or in quality, or a combination of two or more of these dimensions in relation to age, sex, size, and cultural background. It should be noted that there are variations within some parts of the country where quality such as "nasal twang" would be considered acceptable but not in other parts. Racial backgrounds should also be taken into consideration in such judgments, as suggested by Awan and Mueller (1996), who state that there are observed differences among white, African American, and Hispanic children in pitch and range. They caution the speech pathologist to exercise discretion when assessing these characteristics in children of different racial backgrounds.

A voice disorder can interfere with successful communication in at least two ways. The presence of a voice disorder tends to attract adverse attention to the voice and by so doing can get in the way of the intended message. Second, vocal distortion caused by the disorder itself might interfere with the intelligibility of the message.

The essential parts of the voice-producing mechanism or system are the lungs, vocal folds, and resonators. These are responsible for pitch, loudness, and quality of voice.

Pitch

The air from the lungs causes the vocal folds to vibrate. If they vibrate slowly, the pitch is perceived as lower, and if rapidly, the pitch is perceived as higher.

Have you ever heard a female voice that sounded like a man's? Or, conversely, have you ever heard a male voice that sounded like that of a woman? Most of us have. Our immediate impression is that the voice we are hearing is not appropriate in *pitch* for the age and gender of the speaker. Such a voice draws adverse attention to itself. Another circumstance is when pitch "breaks." Now it's high and suddenly it's low. This is frequently associated with adolescent males who are undergoing "voice change." A very unusual case of pitch is heard in a person who seemingly has two pitches, used simultaneously.

Loudness

Loudness, like pitch, is a perceptual judgment. A child whose only problem is a voice that is described as too loud or too soft is rarely enrolled in speech therapy. However, sometimes loudness is one factor of a larger problem, most notably increased loudness levels related to vocal abuse (explained later in this chapter). It should also be noted that voices that are too soft or too loud are sometimes indicative of hearing loss.

Quality Related to Vocal Fold Action

Whereas a normal voice can be described as pleasant (or at least not unpleasant) and smooth sounding, poor vocal quality may be described as hoarse, harsh, rough, breathy, strident, grating, too low or too high in pitch, or monotonous. Such characteristics are related to vocal fold action.

Quality Related to Resonance

Sound produced by the vocal folds travels through the various cavities of the throat and head. Although all of us have similar structures, individual differences in them make each unique. Therefore, the resonation of our voices is also different, which makes for differences in voice quality among speakers. Most problems of resonance are related to the perceived degree of nasality present in the voice. In voices too highly nasalized there is too much vocal tone passing through the nasal cavity. In the English language only the sounds "m," "n," and "ng" are to be positively resonated nasally. When there is too little nasal resonation, the speaker sounds as though he or she is talking with a head cold.

What Are the Causes of Voice Disorders?

To attempt to present a full description of all the possible organic and functional causes of voice disorders in children would go far beyond the scope of this book. For our purposes here it is best for the classroom teacher to think of the disorders that can occur in terms of two normal voice production processes: phonation and resonance.

Phonation

Phonation refers to the production of sound by the vibrations of the vocal folds and is a complex process. Humans have two vocal folds, which are housed in the larynx (the Adam's apple, or voice box, in the neck) and lie side by side in a front-to-back position. As we use our voices, healthy vocal folds vibrate, coming together smoothly along the length of their surfaces at the midline, separating, and then coming together again. This action is very rapid, so rapid that the naked eye cannot follow the individual movements. The rapidity of vibration is determined by the air pressure coming from the lungs beneath the vocal folds, the tension of the vocal folds, the mass of the vocal folds, and the length of the vocal folds. The rate or frequency of vibration is the physical correlate to what we subjectively perceive as pitch. If the frequency is slower than normal, we perceive the speaker's pitch as being low, whereas if the rate is faster than normal, we perceive the pitch as being high. If the vocal folds do not come together smoothly along their edges, the quality of the voice (as related to phonation) will be judged abnormal and words like "hoarse," "husky," "breathy," or "strident," may be used to describe it. The energy source for phonation or voice production is the air that we exhale. This air stream must be steady and sufficient. For normal respiration and vocal fold movement to occur, there must be normal neural and muscular activity. Any condition that interferes with the neural impulses directed to the respiratory or laryngeal muscles, or with the muscular activity itself, will result in a vocal disturbance. One such condition that teachers will encounter is cerebral palsy, which is discussed further in Chapter 8.

Voice disorders can result from vocal abuse and vocal misuse; trauma to the larynx resulting from accidents or medical procedures, such as intubation (a tube is passed between the vocal folds in the larynx into the trachea); congenital mal-formations of the larynx; organic diseases or conditions; tumors; emotional prob-lems; or functional causes, such as the imitation of poor speech models, when no known organic causes exist. In this discussion we will assume that neural and muscular activities are normal and will focus on phonation. Following is a discus-sion of the terms that a teacher will most likely hear in reference to the school-age child or youth who has a phonatory voice disorder.

Abuse and Misuse of the Voice

Vocal abuse and misuse involve improper use of the vocal mechanism. Examples include screaming, yelling, shrieking, loud talking, excessive use of the voice, grunt-ing, and abrupt initiation of voicing (hard glottal attack) (Andrews, 1991). Also loud forced laughter, loud speaking or singing, loud talking that is necessary in a noisy environment, unusual use of the voice to make animal or machine-like sounds, coughing, throat clearing, and smoking can constitute vocal abuse or misuse.

Perhaps the reader has been involved in some of these behaviors at one time or another after which you were temporarily hoarse. For some, such behaviors may cause a voice disorder.

Children in their excitement or in their desire to control may scream at times. Screaming loudly and too often can most certainly have long-lasting effects on their voices. Such activity may be related to a child's personality or environment. The very aggressive child is more apt to yell and speak loudly to command atten-tion. Children can learn to be loud. Loud parents, loud children! Sibling-rivalry or a television that is constantly turned on far too loudly can be factors contributing to loud speech and vocal abuse. Additionally, as Andrews and Summers (1988) point out, asthma, allergies, chemically induced irritation, vocally demanding activities, and respiratory disorders are all potential contributors to vocal abuse.

The term *vocal hygiene* refers to the proper use of the voice. Teachers who dis-courage screaming and yelling while encouraging children to speak at a conversa-tional level with their "inside" voices are not only achieving a quieter, more learning-conducive environment but are also encouraging vocal hygiene. To be even more helpful, classroom teachers might consider consulting with a speech-language pathologist and incorporating a unit on vocal hygiene into the health or science curriculum. It would be a good idea for staff members at the school who direct activities such as cheerleading, sports, drama, and singing to consult with the speech-language pathologist on the use and misuse of the voice. For example, a cheerleading sponsor might wish to invite the speech-language pathologist to teach a lesson on how to cheer without abusing the voice. This writer has had occasion to deal clinically with cheerleaders who have come to the clinic com-plaining of hoarse voice and discomfort particularly after sports events.

Vocal Polyps

Vocal abuse can lead to the development of polyps on the vocal folds. The symp-toms are frequently hoarseness and breathiness. Not only abuse but also other conditions cited earlier (i.e., asthma, allergies, etc.) can be causative factors. Vocal polyps can occur on one or both vocal folds. If discovered early enough, vocal therapy is the procedure of choice. If they are permitted to continue, the chances are greater that surgery will be necessary. The physician (otolaryngologist) is the one to make the diagnosis as to the presence and possible cause of the polyps, and whether or not surgical removal or vocal therapy is indicated. Sometimes both surgical removal and vocal therapy are recommended. Whether polyps are removed by surgery or through vocal therapy, vocal habits causing the polyps must be eliminated to prevent their recurrence.

Vocal Nodules
Abuse of the voice may also cause the development of vocal nodules, sometimes referred to as *singer's nodules* or *screamer's nodules*. They are similar to vocal cord polyps but are firmer and do not respond to vocal rest. Fortunately in children the nodules are most frequently eliminated with voice therapy and modification of the child's voice behavior.

Juvenile Papillomas
Papillomas are the most frequently seen noncancerous tumors in children even as young as 1 year of age and are caused by a virus (Berkow, 1997). They grow rapidly and can cause hoarseness and may obstruct the airway. They are removed surgically or by laser vaporization. Total vocal rest might be required for 7 to 10 days following removal. If this is the case, the classroom teacher has an important role to play in providing emotional support and encouragement to the child.

Contact Ulcers
This also is a condition that results from vocal abuse and is frequently seen in individuals who use their voices a great deal. The ulcer is a sore on the mucous membrane that covers the cartilages to which the vocal cords are attached (Berkow, 1997). The writer has had personal acquaintance with a contact ulcer in adult life. Apprehended early by a speech-language pathologist with stroboscopy and further examination by an otolaryngologist who recommended vocal therapy, the ulcer was cleared up in clinical sessions of vocal therapy within 2 months.

Puberphonia or Mutational Falsetto
The term *mutation* refers to the lowering of a person's pitch that normally occurs during puberty. This process takes the male about 3 to 6 months to complete, at which time the voice is pitched on the average about one octave lower. Girls' voices lower about three to four semitones. Andrews and Summers (1988) suggested that for the male the growth of facial hair, which occurs during the latter stages of pubertal maturation, can be used as a guideline for determining whether maturationally a boy's pitch should have become lower. The majority of youth pass through this stage with no problems. However, although the vocal mechanism develops, occasionally the voice does not fully develop into that of a normal sounding adult. The terms *puberphonia* or *mutational falsetto* are used to describe the problem of unnaturally high pitch that is not a result of hormonal disorders. Therapy is generally successful in a relatively short period of time.

On occasion the vocal mechanism does not develop appropriately in relation to the other development that is taking place. The writer has dealt with such a case clinically. The case history of Ralph at the end of the chapter explains the circumstances in some detail.

Resonance

Air and the laryngeal tone (the sound that is produced by the vocal folds) travel up into the throat, mouth, and nasal cavity. The sizes and shapes of these three structures and the way in which they are connected to each other change the way the laryngeal tone sounds. This change process is referred to as *resonance.* You can easily demonstrate how the size and shape of structures influence resonance by taking several 16-ounce bottles, leaving one empty and filling the others with varying amounts of water, blowing across the tops of the bottles much as one would play the flute, and listening to the various pitch sounds that are produced. The most common resonance disorders involve the way the nasal cavity (nose) is connected to the oral cavity (mouth). The *palate* is the structure in the mouth that serves as the roof of the mouth and the floor of the nasal cavity. If you place your tongue on the roof of your mouth immediately behind your top teeth and slowly move your tongue backward along the palate, you will note that approximately the first two-thirds of the palate feels hard (because there is bone beneath the layers of soft tissue), and then the palate becomes soft (there is no longer any bony tissue). The bony two-thirds of the palate is referred to as the *hard palate* and the soft one-third as the *soft palate* or *velum.* The velum is composed partially of muscles, which allow the velum to stretch upward and backward to the back wall of the throat. (Look in a mirror, say "aah," and note this movement.) As the velum moves, the back and side walls of the throat (or pharynx) move slightly forward and inward to meet the velum. These movements together cause the nasal cavity to be shut off from the mouth. A teacher may hear this opening between the nose and mouth referred to as the *velopharyngeal* port and the involved structures referred to as the *velopharyngeal mechanism* ("velo" from "velum"—soft palate; "pharyngeal" from "pharynx"—throat). If there is a problem, a child may be said to have velopharyngeal incompetency or insufficiency. The cause of velopharyngeal incompetency may be functional (no organic cause can be found) or organic (structural or physiological causes can be found).

Hypernasality

When the nasal cavity cannot be sufficiently shut off from the oral cavity due to velopharyngeal incompetency, the voice sounds *nasal.* Why? Because some sounds other than the truly nasal sounds "m," "n," and "ng" are also delivered through the nose. Sometimes, when the lack of adequate velopharyngeal closure is very pronounced, the listener might actually hear the air escaping from the nose of the speaker. To prevent this, the speaker may try to close the nostrils. In extreme cases the hypernasality is accompanied by sound distortions, substitutions, or omissions in an attempt to overcome the problem. This in turn can affect the intelligibility of speech.

Hypernasality may occur as a result of a cleft palate or a submucous cleft. These will be discussed further in a later section on cleft palate. Hypernasality may come as a result of removal of adenoids that creates a hiatus between the velum and the pharyngeal wall. The case history of Cheryl Mae at the end of this chapter illustrates this problem.

The speech-language pathologist dealing with the child, the parents, and the classroom teacher will call upon specialized medical assistance for guidance about problems of hypernasality. Structural problems cannot always be determined adequately through the usual visual inspection procedures. The new imaging techniques, however, provide additional help in the medical diagnosis. It should be noted as well that a developing hypernasality may be due to causes other than structural, which need medical evaluation.

Hyponasality

Less common than hypernasality, hyponasality (or denasality) occurs when the nasal passages are occluded. This may be due to nasal congestion associated with respiratory infections or allergies; enlarged adenoids, which fill up the space between the soft palate and walls of the throat so that air and sound cannot enter the nasal cavity; tumors; congenital anomalies; or changes in the nasal structures due to accidents that prevent sounds and air from entering the nasal cavity. By necessity, the child who is hyponasal due to organic problems will be a mouth-breather. Treatment may consist of decongestants and other medical-surgical procedures.

Can Voice Problems Be Related to Other Conditions?

The answer is yes. The voice problem itself may be a symptom of a more serious and complicated medical condition. Therefore, the speech-language pathologist generally insists that the person with a voice problem be examined by a physician (preferably an otolaryngologist) before initiating any vocal therapy. The otolaryngologist is specialized in the treatment of ear, nose, and throat problems. He or she can view the vocal folds through a procedure called indirect larnygoscopy with the use of a laryngeal mirror. If there is need to examine further, more advanced techniques such as rigid endoscopy, stroboscopy, or other imaging procedures are used (Colton & Casper, 1990). Several conditions can be associated with similar sounding voices, but the otolaryngologist's report will give the speech-language pathologist the results of the examination and any medical recommendations. Various problems can be significant in voice disorders, such as congenital anomalies of the laryngeal mechanism, psychiatric conditions, tumors, infections, endocrine disorders, hearing loss, cerebral palsy, nasal obstructions, obstructive sleep apnea syndrome, trauma, and lesions (Andrews, 1995). Depending on the problem, medical or surgical intervention, voice therapy, or a combination of services may be appropriate. The best care is given to the child when the physician, speech-language pathologist, classroom teacher, and parents work together. The physician's report might suggest that no therapy be undertaken but that other action should be taken either medically or surgically. However, if therapy is indicated, the medical report and periodic reexamination can be the baseline for determining progress in the therapy program. Thus, it is very important for classroom teachers to be aware of children with possible voice disorders and refer them to a speech-language pathologist for assessment.

How Is the Voice Assessed and Evaluated?

Assessment

Assessment implies obtaining as many objective measures as warranted of the child's voice. This can be accomplished by the speech-language pathologist by rating the voice of the child on the several dimensions of quality, pitch, and loudness. It might also involve recording the child's voice several times over a period of several weeks to ensure that what is being heard as a voice disorder is not a temporary aberration due to a cold, allergy, et cetera. This preliminary screening approach can be supplemented by using available published tests and indices directed toward voice assessment such as the systematic protocol developed by Pindzola (1999) that samples vocal pitch, loudness, quality, breath features, and rate/rhythm, or an index of vocal behavior that yields performance ranges by age and gender by Johnston and Umberger (1998). These instruments and similar ones provide a formal frame of reference for deriving data on the voice of the child.

Not to be overlooked is hearing screening and possible indepth testing, if necessary, of the child with a vocal disorder. If hearing loss exists, it could be a factor in the development of voice quality.

Research continues in various institutions in the United States and elsewhere aimed at learning more about the nature and consequences of voice disorders, such as that conducted by Heylen and colleagues (1998), who analyzed voice range profiles of children according to 11 characteristics of frequency, intensity, and morphology. The point of the research was to demonstrate how a voice range profile can be used in screening children for vocal disorders or to assess quantitatively the effectiveness of voice therapy.

Evaluation

If the results of assessment indicate a need for further inquiry, the speech-language pathologist will want to obtain a medical history and additional information from the child, parent, and teachers regarding behaviors associated with vocal abuse. If the evaluation of these data indicates that the child does indeed have abnormal vocal aspects, parents must be consulted about referral of the child to an otolaryngologist or perhaps other medical or psychological specialists for further evaluation and possible intervention and guidance.

Measuring vocal characteristics is tremendously important. However, determining quantitatively the psychosocial impact of a voice disorder is yet another matter. Until recently only few attempts at quantification of psychosocial impact in the area of voice disorders have been undertaken. Jacobson and colleagues (1997) took on the challenge and carried out an investigation through which they developed an index that provided information concerning the psychosocial effects of a voice handicap.

What Is Involved in Voice Therapy?

Have you ever made a recording of your voice and played it back? What a shock! That doesn't sound like my voice! True, it doesn't sound like you to your ears. But if the recording is a good one, it probably really sounds like you to other listeners. Why the difference? The difference lies in the fact that we do not hear ourselves as others hear us because we are producing the voice. Our voice is heard by others as it passes from our mouths out into the room. Our voice is heard by ourselves in at least a couple of ways. First, we hear our own voice as it travels through the tissue between the vocal folds and the ear. Second, we hear our own voice as it travels out of our mouth and is picked up by our external ears. (It is interesting to note also that the arrival time of the voice traveling the tissue route is slightly different from that which is delivered out of the mouth and picked up as "side tone" by our ears.)

Because many of the problems of voice seen in children are a result of vocal abuse, there are some steps that can be taken to reduce and eventually eliminate it. These are undertaken by the child, the parent, the teacher, and the speech-language pathologist. It has been suggested that even individuals who are in contact with the child in other capacities might be of help.

What are the steps that can be taken? Frequently voice therapy begins with an emphasis on the development of listening skills. The intent is to train the child to hear his or her own voice and to learn to recognize those aspects of it that need to be changed. It is a discrimination task. This can be done in several ways: with isolated vowels, words, phrases, and sentences. Auditory stimulation is fundamental in attempting to help build new vocal behavior. The child must have a model to follow, whether it be for pitch, loudness, or other characteristics. There should be praise for successful attempts throughout the process that reinforces the child's efforts.

When indicated, a program of accounting for the number of instances of abuse should be put into place. This calls for counting the times the child engages in vocal abuse. For this to be effective, many individuals should be involved. The child, of course, should be alerted to keep track of the abuses in particular situations such as the playground or at home. Likewise, the assistance of parents is vital in the home situation. Surely the classroom teacher is in a strategic position to determine within a span of time the abuses heard and also to encourage the child to participate in speaking activities. The speech-language pathologist also is very helpful here within a limited time frame. The object is to tally the number of abuses in various situations over a certain time period, perhaps several weeks or perhaps a month, and after the predetermined length of time to ascertain whether, with proper counseling, the number of abuses is being reduced. Optimally the abuses will be eliminated eventually. It is very important, as previously stated, to give the child positive reinforcement for successful attempts to reduce the instances of abuse.

In the attempt to reduce vocal abuse the child should be taught how his or her vocal mechanism works. If the child has a visual image of the operation of the voice mechanism, this should help in understanding how damage is done to the mechanism through abuse.

Another very general approach in helping high-strung, loud talking, yelling children to improve their use of voice is to help them learn to relax. This is not accomplished very well by merely suggesting relaxation but by demonstrating the difference between bodily tension and a relaxed body and between a tense voice and a voice that is relaxed.

Various books, programs, methods, techniques, and materials have been developed through the years by speech-language pathologists focusing specifically on voice problems (Harris & Harris, 1997; Johnson, 1995; Agnello & Garcia, 1990; Boone, 1980; Case, 1996; Johnston & Umberger, 1996). It should be emphasized, however, that although there are some general procedures to follow, as outlined in published materials, the speech-language pathologist will tailor therapy sessions to the individual needs of the child. The classroom teacher, although busy with the responsibilities of an entire classroom, must be kept aware of what is taking place with the child or children in her classroom undergoing therapy. With this information the teacher can play a vital role in monitoring vocal behavior and reinforcing the work of the speech-language pathologist.

What Is Cleft Palate?

Many teachers-in-training raise a number of questions about cleft palate. What is cleft palate? How often does cleft palate occur? What causes a cleft lip or cleft palate? Can cleft palate and cleft lip be corrected? How does a cleft lip and/or cleft palate affect a child's speech? What should I as a teacher or a student preparing to become a teacher know about cleft palate and cleft lip? This section will provide some information to address these questions.

A cleft, which can involve the lip and/or palate, is an opening in these structures due to their failure to close or fuse during early development of the fetus. These structures normally are fused sometime within the first 3 months of fetal development. Failure to develop properly may result in a cleft of one or both sides of the upper lip, a cleft of the palate alone, of the lip alone, or of both palate and lip. The extent or severity of a cleft is variable as well. In some instances it may be relatively small and restricted only to the lip or palate, whereas in others it may be extensive and involve both lip and hard and soft palates.

Many causes without scientific basis are attributed to cleft lip and palate. Legend has it that a baby born with a cleft lip or palate is punishment for parents who are in disfavor of the Almighty, or that the child is not really wanted. These and other such attributions are myths. However, scientists are still seeking answers that are based in fact. Currently the best indications are that this anomaly in development is genetically related and seems to follow in families. It may be that the two variables of genetic predisposition toward a cleft and the environment provided a fetus together caused this maldevelopment.

One of every 700 newborns has some form of cleft lip and/or palate, the fourth most common birth defect (Beverly-Ducker, 1992). The frequency of occurrence is related to race and gender. Incidence estimates vary as follows: whites, approximately 1 in 750 to 1,000 births; for blacks, approximately 1 in 1,900 to 3,000 births; and for Asians about 1 in 500 births. Clefts are seen more frequently in boys than in girls (McWilliams, 1986).

Correction of cleft palate is best accomplished by an interdisciplinary team composed of representatives from surgery, dentistry, nursing, orthodontics, prosthodontics, psychology, medical social work, speech-language pathology, and audiology. Medical and dental correction involves surgical repair and the fitting of prosthetic appliances. The surgical approach calls for specialized surgical procedures. In some instances, depending upon the nature and severity of the cleft, several operations over many years may be necessary. In those cases in which surgery is inappropriate or has not culminated in a complete closure, a prosthetic appliance called an *obturator* is used. The obturator fills the opening created by the maldevelopment. It is also possible to fit missing teeth (a not uncommon problem) onto an obturator. As a child grows, the obturator must be replaced periodically. Contraindications to an obturator include severe mental retardation, uncooperative parents or child, or an extremely poor dental situation.

For some children, early medical treatment and a good program of speech-language stimulation in infancy will correct most adverse effects on speech by the time a child begins school. Harding and Grunwell (1998) point out, however, that surgery is quite effective in eliminating some cleft palate speech characteristics but not as effective in eliminating others. Although for many children a cleft lip and palate may affect speech adversely, surgical repair and prosthetic devices help to provide the structures necessary for acceptable speech. The classroom teacher can be crucial in the early detection and referral of these children to the speech-language pathologist. Early detection and a good program of therapy that involves the parents are of great importance. Blakely and Brockman (1995) describe the success they achieved by age 5 with young children with cleft palates. The goal of normalcy was set for oral-nasal balance, articulation, and hearing. They achieved 93 percent normalcy in both oral-nasal balance and normal developmental articulation and 98 percent for normal hearing in at least one ear. Their study demonstrates vividly the positive effects of multidisciplinary and parental involvement in habilitating children with speech and hearing problems caused by cleft palate.

It has been suggested by some that children with cleft palates are stigmatized by their speech during early years of life. Here again is an opportunity for the classroom teacher to play a key role in helping the child to be accepted by eliciting the support of the other children.

An interesting study was made by Bressman et al. (1998), who administered instruments to parents of children with cleft palate to determine quality of life, social support, and family life characteristics. The results obtained indicated that the overall quality of life is very good for their cleft palate patients; social integration appeared to be no different from their non–cleft palate population; and the presence of a child with cleft palate had no severe long-term impact on family life. These findings are in agreement with some of the early studies reported in the literature.

Cleft palate speech may be characterized by articulatory errors. Some omissions, substitutions, and insertions might be associated with the physical anomaly and of course there might be some that appear quite apart from the physical aberration just as they do in children without clefts. Some might be sounds that do not occur in the English language, such as the glottal stop. Along with all of this there might be nasal emission of air, and facial grimaces, all of which are compensatory efforts to trap the air escaping through the nose to allow better sound production.

As for cognitive and linguistic features of children with cleft palate, early studies indicated that children with cleft palates demonstrate a slight but not significant reduction in language skills. Broen and colleagues (1998), in a comparison of the cognitive and linguistic development of two groups of children, one with cleft palates and the other without, found that *both groups* were *within normal range* as measured by appropriate developmental mental and physical instruments, mean length of words, and words acquired by 24 months. However, they did find significant differences between the two groups in relation to some aspects of the variables studied. In cognitive development the differences were related to verbal as opposed to nonverbal performance, to hearing status at 12 months, and to velopharyngeal adequacy.

Some children with clefts also have congenital and/or other problems. Blakely and Brockman (1995) report that in their 4-year study of children with cleft palates there were 15 who also showed the effects of congenital and/or psychosocial abnormalities including fetal alcohol syndrome, severely dysfunctional families, Prader-Will syndrome, and pulmonary stenosis.

It is very important that classroom teachers are fully aware of the implications of cosmetic, speech, and related problems the child with cleft palate might face. Close liaison with parents, the speech-language pathologist, and children about these problems is much to be desired.

For a more detailed explanation of cleft palate and cleft lip and the approaches used in habilitation, the reader might wish to consult the well-developed literature in this field, including such sources as Bzoch (1997) and Moller and Starr (1993).

Case Histories

Ralph

The case of Ralph is unusual. Ralph was referred to the speech-language and hearing clinic because of a vocal pitch problem. The referral source was concerned that his pitch was too high for a 17-year-old boy. This writer was the clinician who made the initial assessment. Ralph was a well-developed young man, a high achiever academically, and a varsity football player at his high school. The level of his vocal pitch came as somewhat of a surprise. Examination showed that his habitual pitch was indeed too high for his age and gender. Also his vocal range was restricted. An attempt to see whether or not he could extend his vocal range gave evidence that he could not do so. If I had not seen Ralph but had only heard his voice, I would have believed I was listening to the voice of a young boy or girl not having reached puberty.

Ralph was referred to an otolaryngologist for a medical examination. The following week the physician's report reached the clinic. It stated that Ralph had an underdeveloped laryngeal mechanism that would most likely never develop any further. What action was taken? No vocal therapy program was appropriate, but Ralph and his parents were counseled about his status. Positive features of his situation were emphasized, that is, his success as a student and athlete and his overall good physical development. Although the pitch of his voice did call adverse attention to itself, it was offset by his affable nature and his achievements.

Cheryl Mae

Cheryl Mae, age 8 years, was referred to this writer because of a severe voice problem. She had an extreme case of hypernasality that developed following the removal of tonsils and adenoids. On initial evaluation it became evident that she was not going to be able to modify her quality to a level of acceptability. She was referred to an otolaryngologist, who made x-ray films of her throat. They showed a gap that defied velopharyngeal closure. The first course of action was a surgical procedure to assist in velopharyngeal closure. This at first showed promise for the nasality problem, with the help of a speech-language pathologist. But after a few months the therapy yielded no more progress. The otolaryngologist recommended a pharyngeal flap operation. This was accomplished, and again vocal therapy was undertaken in Cheryl's home town with the local speech-language pathologist. Some improvement was noted, but the speech quality was still hypernasal. After some months of therapy, Cheryl Mae and her parents decided to try to monitor her speech without the aid of her speech-language pathologist.

This writer had the opportunity to speak with Cheryl Mae some years later and could see that the pharyngeal flap operation and subsequent therapy had yielded some positive effects on her voice quality. Many years later the writer again spoke with Cheryl Mae (now aged 40) and was delighted to see that her voice quality had improved considerably through the years.

Jonie

One of Jonie's teachers referred her to the speech-language pathologist because her voice was very husky and low pitched. Upon assessment by the speech-language pathologist, it was learned that Jonie, then a junior in high school, was a very outgoing girl who talked constantly. To further complicate the picture, Jonie was a cheerleader and yelled incessantly at sports events. The case history revealed that on many mornings following a game she was literally voiceless. There was little question but that she was in trouble already, and without help she would most certainly be even more deeply in trouble with her voice.

The speech-language pathologist consulted with Jonie's parents about the seriousness of the situation. The parents agreed to have Jonie seen by an otolaryngologist to determine whether medical or surgical treatment was necessary. Fortunately neither was, but the otolaryngologist described Jonie's swollen and reddened vocal folds and warned of the danger of developing polyps or vocal nodules if the yelling continued. The otolaryngologist put Jonie on vocal rest for 3 weeks: no yelling, no talking, no whispering. Jonie continued at games as a cheerleader, but strictly without voice.

Following the period of vocal rest, Jonie's voice was much improved; only a slight trace of huskiness remained. A program of vocal hygiene was outlined for Jonie, and she met regularly with the speech-language pathologist for its implementation. The latest word is that therapy is moving along well and that Jonie, although still a very outgoing girl, is seeing the wisdom of being much more careful about not abusing her voice.

Richard

Richard was a fourth-grader who had been born with an extensive cleft of both lip and palate. He had undergone several operations as a preschooler, and both the lip and palate had been repaired. Prior to his direct work in the speech therapy class, he had received no other special help because he lived in a rural area where public school speech therapy had been unavailable prior to the enactment of PL 94-142. Thus, Richard was 9 years old before he had any opportunity to improve his speech. Unfortunately, unlike some children with repaired clefts, his speech, even with the excellent palatal repair, was nasal to the point of being unintelligible at times. He was shy and old enough to be quite embarrassed about his unsuccessful attempts at communicating with his teacher and his classmates. To make matters worse, he was the butt of many wisecracks made by some pupils, despite the classroom teacher's attempts to stop them.

Richard's work with the speech-language pathologist was a bright spot in the day for both Richard and his clinician. He not only eagerly accepted help but also made excellent progress in the development of better articulation and a voice that was considerably less nasal. His classroom teacher worked intelligently and enthusiastically with Richard and the speech-language pathologist. She maintained a "transfer sheet" of sounds (set up by the clinician) that Richard could be expected to produce successfully in the classroom. Richard seemed to be gaining more confidence each day, and after a year of special help he had made substantial progress. It appeared also that his fellow pupils were including him more in their play and accepting him much better. He obviously was thinking more highly of himself, and they were seemingly regarding him more favorably.

One day the following autumn a youngster was referred to the clinician by the kindergarten teacher. It was John, Richard's younger brother. Evaluation quickly revealed that John had cleft palate speech as well. The only difference was that John had a perfect speech mechanism—no cleft lip—no cleft palate! He had simply learned Richard's cleft palate speech in his 5 years at home. A real challenge!

Summary

Causes of Voice Problems

- Learning faulty speech patterns
- Vocal abuse
- Allergies
- Maldevelopment of the vocal mechanism
- Frequent infections
- Trauma
- Emotional problems
- Vocal nodules and tumors
- Vocal changes in puberty

Some Important Points to Remember

- Voice problems can interfere with successful communication.
- Early detection of voice problems is important.
- The parents, classroom teacher, speech-language pathologist, and physician are important for successful vocal therapy.
- Surveys show that 6 to 9 percent of children have voice disorders.
- Based upon frequency of occurrence, children with voice disorders are under-represented in the caseloads of speech-language pathologists.
- Examination by a physician (otolaryngologist) is frequently indicated for children with voice problems.
- There are disorders of pitch, loudness, and quality (related to both phonation and resonance).
- Hyponasality refers to too little nasal resonance.
- Hypernasality refers to too much nasal resonance.
- Vocal assessment involves a case history and voice examination by the speech-language pathologist, and frequently a medical examination.
- Cleft palate and cleft lip can cause voice and articulation disorders.

"Do"s and "Don't"s for Teachers

"Do"s

- Be aware of children with unusual sounding voices and refer them to a speech-language pathologist.
- Learn from the speech-language pathologist the nature of a child's disorder and how you can help.
- Reinforce the work of the speech-language pathologist.
- Create an atmosphere of acceptance and understanding in the classroom for the child with a voice disorder.

"Don't"s

- Do not attempt to correct a voice disorder except as instructed by a speech-language pathologist.

Referral Resources

- Speech-language pathologist
- Otolaryngologist
- Allergist
- Psychologist
- Audiologist
- Cleft palate team

Self Test

True or False:

1. The voice sometimes reflects the speaker's emotions and physical health.   _____

2. A hypernasal voice is one with too much nasality.   _____

3. A hyponasal voice is one with too little nasality.   _____

4. An acceptable figure for prevalence of voice disorders in children is from 25 to 30 percent.   _____

5. There is some concern that children with voice disorders have been under-represented in the caseloads of speech-language pathologists.   _____

6. Voice problems may be indicative of medical conditions.   _____

7. The majority of youth pass through puberty without any serious voice problems.   _____

8. The throat, mouth, and nasal cavities contribute insignificantly to the resonance characteristics of the voice.   _____

9. *Resonance* refers to the production of sound by the vibrations of the vocal folds.   _____

10. When making an assessment of voice, the speech-language pathologist is concerned with checking quality, pitch, and loudness.   _____

11. We hear our voices as others hear them.   _____

12. Children with voice disorders due to vocal abuse may need to be evaluated relative to their psychological and emotional adjustment.   _____

13. *Vocal hygiene* refers to therapy for voice disorders.   _____

14. The causes for cleft palate and cleft lip have yet to be firmly established.   _____

15. Cleft palate usually occurs sometime between birth and the end of the first year.   _____

16. Clefts vary considerably in type and severity.   _____

17. Where there is a cleft lip, there is always a cleft palate.   _____

18. Both hard and soft palates may be cleft in some babies.   _____

19. Figures show that the frequency of cleft palates is considerably higher among blacks than among Asians.   _____

20. Rarely is surgical repair an option for a child with cleft lip and cleft palate.   _____

21. A prosthetic appliance called an obturator is sometimes used for filling the space created by a cleft.   _____

22. The speech of children with cleft palate is frequently hyponasal.   _____

23. More boys are born with a cleft palate than girls.   _____

24. A multidisciplinary team effort is indicated for a child with a cleft palate and lip.   _____

25. An obturator is an appliance used in cases of cleft lip.   _____

References

Agnello, V., & Garcia, C. (1990). *Vocal rehabilitation.* Austin, TX: Pro-Ed.

Andrews, M. (1995). Pediatric voice problems associated with other conditions. In *Manual of voice treatment.* (vol. 3) (p. 172). San Diego, CA: Singular Publishing Group.

Andrews, M., & Summers, R. (1988). *Vocal therapy for adolescents.* Boston: College-Hill/Little, Brown.

Awan, S., & Mueller, P. (1996). Speaking fundamental frequency characteristics of white, African American, and Hispanic kindergartners. *Journal of Speech and Hearing Research, 39,* 573.

Berkow, R. (Ed). (1997). "Ear, nose and throat problems." Whitehouse Station, NJ: Merck Research Laboratories. In *The Merck manual of medical information.*

Beverly-Ducker, K. (1992). Cleft palate-craniofacial groups. *ASHA, 34,* (4), 56.

Blakely, R., & Brockman, J. (1995). Normal speech and hearing by age 5 as a goal for children with cleft palate: A demonstration project. *American Journal of Speech-Language Pathology, 4,* 25.

Boone, D. (1980). The Boone voice program for children. Austin, TX: Pro-Ed.

Bressmann, T., Sader, R., Ravens-Sieberer, U., Zeilhofer, H.-F., & Horch, H.-H. (1998). Normality despite cleft palate: Quality of life, social support, and family life in adolescent and adult patients. Amsterdam, The Netherlands: *Program and Abstract Book.* 24th IALP Congress, *35,* 181.

Broen, P., Devers, M., Doyle S., Prouty, J., & Moller, K. (1998). Acquisition of linguistic and cognitive skills by children with cleft palate. *Journal of Speech, Language, and Hearing Research, 41,* 676.

Bzoch, K. (Ed). (1997). *Communicative disorders related to cleft lip and palate.* (3rd ed.). Austin, TX: Pro-Ed.

Case, J. (1996). *Clinical management of voice disorders.* Austin, TX: Pro-Ed.

Colton, R., & Casper, J. (1990). *Understanding voice problems.* Baltimore, MD: Williams and Wilkins.

Harding, A., & Grunwell, P. (1998). Active versus passive cleft-type speech characteristics. *International Journal of Language and Communication, 33,* 329.

Harris, H., & Harris, S. (1997). *The voice clinic handbook.* London: Whurr.

Heylen, L., Wuyts, F., Mertens, F., De Bodt, M., Pattyn, J., Croux, C., & Van de Heyning, P. (1998). Evaluation of the vocal performance of children using a voice range profile index. *Journal of Speech, Language, and Hearing Research, 41,* 232.

Jacobson, B., Johnson, A., Grywalski, C., Silbergleit, A., Jacobson, G., Benninger, M., & Newman, C. (1997). The voice of handicap index (VHI): Development and validation. *American Journal of Speech-Language Pathology, 6,* 66.

Johnson, S. (1995). *Vocal abuse reduction program.* Austin, TX: Pro-Ed.

Johnston, R., & Umberger, F. (1996). The voice companion. East Moline, IL: LinguiSystems.

Johnston, R., & Umberger, F. (1998). *The voice index.* East Moline, IL: LinguiSystems.

McWilliams, B. (1986). Cleft palate. In G. H. Shames & E. H. Wiig (Eds.), *Human communication disorders* (2nd ed.) (pp. 445–494). Columbus, OH: Merrill.

Moller, K., & Starr, C. (1993). *Interdisciplinary issues and treatment for clinicians by clinicians.* Austin, TX: Pro-Ed.

Pindzola, A. (1999). Voice assessment protocol for children and adults. East Aurora, NY: Slosson.

Wilson, D. K. (1987). *Voice problems of children* (3rd ed.). Baltimore, MD: Williams & Wilkins.

Chapter **6**

Hearing and Hearing Loss

Hearing and speech provide the means through which we express and receive ideas, information, and emotions. Speech and language are usually acquired through hearing. Hearing loss can cause individual speech and language systems to be disordered. The resultant communication problems are some of the most serious and challenging to confront a classroom teacher. A significant hearing disability not only signals difficulty understanding the sounds of the environment, but also correlates with serious language, voice, and articulation deficits.

Although it is not common for regular classroom teachers to have the responsibility for children with severe hearing loss, it is likely that many children with moderate to mild losses will be assigned or mainstreamed to a regular classroom for at least part of the school day. Therefore, it is essential that a teacher have a basic understanding of the nature of hearing loss as well as the social, communication, and educational problems that are associated with it.

What Is Sound?

It is difficult for most of us to think of sound as separate from hearing, but they are two distinct concepts. Hearing is like taste, smell, and touch—it is not a physical event; it is a sensation. Sound, therefore, is what our hearing mechanism is engineered to perceive. Accordingly, it is a phenomenon to which our ears are capable of responding, with the implication that sound can be heard if we are present to hear it.

When an object moves in our environment, the disturbed air around the object causes an abnormal air pressure that travels from the site of the object in all directions. If an object vibrates, a series of pressure waves with fluctuations below and above normal air pressure will simulate the vibratory pattern, the back-and-forth motions of the object. These fluctuating pressure changes are called *sound waves*. The strength or power of sound waves correlates with the loudness of the perceived sound. The strength of a sound, therefore, is measured in terms of how much the pressure varies above and below normal atmospheric pressure. This can be referred to as *sound pressure level*.

Sound is also characterized by the rate at which an object vibrates. The slower the cycle of vibrations, the farther apart the sound waves will be spaced. Objects that vibrate at a more rapid rate, or *frequency*, will cause shorter (faster) waves to emanate from the sound source. Therefore, a sound's wavelength always increases as its frequency decreases. Shorter wavelengths, characterized by rapid vibratory rates, are perceived as higher pitched sounds. Longer wavelengths are characterized by slower vibratory rates. Frequency is expressed in cycles per second (cps), also known as hertz (Hz).

Sound *intensity* concerns the strength of the sound waves emanating from an object that has moved or has been set into vibration. The convention for expressing sound intensity is the decibel (dB) scale. The *B* is capitalized in the abbreviated expression in honor of Alexander G. Bell because of his work with sound and hearing. The reference point for describing dB changes is usually zero dB. In measurement of hearing sensitivity this reference typically represents the softest sound we can detect and can be referred to as the *threshold of hearing*. Our upper tolerance for sound intensity is variable, but for practical purposes, any sound level that elicits a painful or tickling sensation in the ears can be considered too intense, and for most of us this occurs between 115 and 140 dB. (See Figure 6-1.)

The psychological correlates of these physical phenomena are loudness for intensity and pitch for frequency. It should be noted that most sounds in our environment are complex in structure. This means that many frequencies with varying intensities are occurring at the same time. Speech is an excellent example of a complex sound.

What Is Normal Hearing?

All sounds are air pressure variations, but some of these variations are beyond our ability to hear. For example, bats generate sounds up to a vibratory rate of 30,000 Hz. The pitch level is so high that it is out of the range of human hearing altogether. There are numerous other sounds, such as certain dog whistles, that possess intensity and frequency characteristics that humans do no have the capability of hearing.

The frequency and intensity boundaries for human hearing are narrow but variable. The lowest audible frequency for most of us is around 15 Hz, which is generally heard as a low pitched rumble and felt as vibrations throughout the body. The upper boundary is generally around 12,000 to 18,000 Hz. The important frequency range for hearing speech is between 300 to 4,000 Hz.

The physical characteristics of sound can be processed by one ear. Why do we have two? The reason is that one ear does not tell us all we want to know about a sound. For example, the location or origin of a particular sound is not easily traced with one ear. Listeners depend on the difference in time for a sound to reach each ear to make these judgments. When one ear is blocked or damaged to the point that hearing is not possible, localizing sound is difficult, if not impossible, particularly in noisy situations.

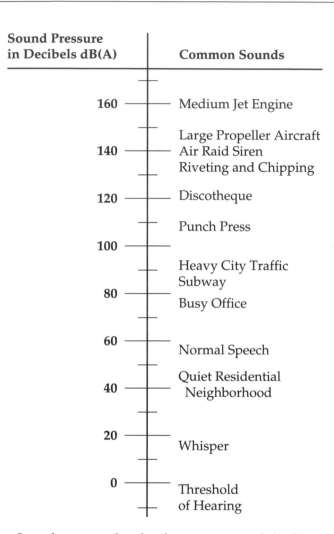

Sound Pressure in Decibels dB(A) | **Common Sounds**

160 — Medium Jet Engine

140 — Large Propeller Aircraft
Air Raid Siren
Riveting and Chipping

120 — Discotheque

Punch Press

100 —

Heavy City Traffic
Subway
80 — Busy Office

60 —
Normal Speech

Quiet Residential
40 — Neighborhood

20 —
Whisper

0 —
Threshold
of Hearing

FIGURE 6–1   Sound pressure levels of common sounds in dB.

How Do We Hear?

The hearing centers in the brain are essentially isolated from the environment. All the important information about sound that gets to the brain is piped in through the ears. Because the brain functions by diverting electrical impulses from one brain cell to another, the information it processes must be delivered in this form. The ears, therefore, must convert the sound stimulus (air pressure fluctuation) into patterns of electrical impulses that transmit essential information about the sound's intensity, frequency, and location. There are three basic steps in the process. First, the

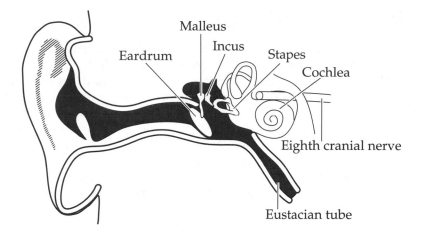

FIGURE 6–2   Structure of the human ear.

atmospheric pressure changes are converted to vibrations. Next, these vibrations are enhanced into stronger vibrations. Last, the vibrations are converted into electrical energy. The three major components of the ear—the outer, middle, and inner ear—are designed to accomplish these objectives. (See Figure 6-2.)

The ear flap, or *pinna*, of the outer ear collects the air pressure fluctuations and channels them through the external ear canal to the eardrum, or *tympanum*. The eardrum also prohibits the free flow of air into the middle ear chamber. As a result, the air pressure differences outside of the middle ear and within the middle ear force the eardrum to bulge in and out in accordance with the air pressure fluctuations impinging upon it. Thereby the eardrum is set into vibration and the air pressure fluctuations are changed in vibratory patterns.

The middle ear is a cavity within the mastoid bone on the side of the skull and is about the size of an ordinary thimble. Normal atmospheric air pressure is maintained within the chamber by a small tube, the *Eustachian tube*, which opens into the throat during the act of swallowing or yawning. The middle ear also houses a chain of three tiny bones, *ossicles*, that connect the eardrum vibrations by mechanical motion to the inner ear. These three bones are called the *malleus, incus,* and *stapes*, and they act as a system of levers to enhance the vibratory energy. The stapes, the last bone in the chain, is attached to a small window-type membrane at the wall of the inner ear (*cochlea*).

The cochlea is filled with fluid and is shaped like a coiled snail shell. The lever action of the middle ear causes pressure changes in the fluid. The movement of the fluid across the nerve endings housed in the inner ear converts the vibrations into electrical impulses. The nerve endings eventually converge into the auditory nerve (there are two nerves, one for each ear), which delivers the electrical impulses to the brain.

How Do We Understand What We Hear?

The process of hearing relies on the brain to interpret the patterns of electrical impulses delivered from each cochlea. However, the meaning that is attached to the sounds of our environment is learned. At birth an infant can detect sounds within the range of human hearing, but sound, in itself, does not carry associated meaning. Within weeks after birth, however, primitive associations among sounds, events, and behaviors are learned. By the end of the first year a normal hearing child understands many words and begins to say them. Children with normal hearing typically develop mature articulation of speech sounds between the ages of 6 and 8. Obviously, hearing plays a critical role in the development of language and speech, because without it a child is incapable of hearing words and thus cannot imitate speech.

How Is Hearing Measured?

The measurement of hearing loss incorporates the concepts of intensity and frequency. This is accomplished by determining the softest sound the ear can detect. It is necessary that the listener be situated in a very quiet room, preferably a sound-treated chamber conforming to nationally accepted standards for eliminating ambient noise. If a stimulus is complex, comprising several frequencies (as does speech), it cannot be determined which component the listener is hearing. Therefore, the sound should be a single frequency of vibration, a *pure tone*. The machine designed to generate these tones is called an *audiometer*. Each pure tone is presented for brief periods of time, with each successive presentation made louder until the listener detects the sound. This procedure is repeated for several different frequencies, usually 125, 250, 500, 1,000, 2,000, 4,000, and 8,000 Hz. The decibel level (intensity) required for hearing at each frequency becomes the threshold of hearing for each frequency. The intensity and frequency for each pure tone that is heard are plotted on a special form called an *audiogram* (Figure 6-3). The symbol "X" indicates responses for the left ear, and "O" signifies responses for the right. Any decibel level below the zero line can be referred to as an *x dB hearing loss* for that frequency. As greater decibel levels are required to hear a particular tone, hearing sensitivity is described as poorer. Accordingly, when lower levels elicit a response, hearing is depicted as better.

The important point is what decibel level of hearing loss at each frequency constitutes a problem for the listener. There is no simple, single answer. A significant loss at any one frequency is not likely to cause a problem. But should several frequencies be affected, a problem is likely. A further question is whether both ears are affected or only one.

Figure 6-3 depicts an audiogram showing hearing loss in both ears. The sensitivity thresholds for the right ear indicate a profound hearing loss causing a significant problem in understanding speech even with the use of a hearing aid. Fortunately, the threshold levels for the left ear are somewhat better, providing a situation in which the listener can perhaps understand speech from the ear when

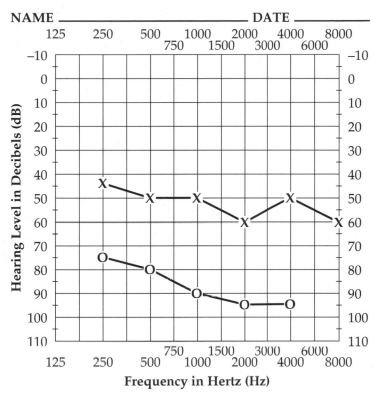

FIGURE 6–3   An audiogram used to plot hearing loss levels.

the signals are loud enough. Roberts, Wallace, and Henderson (1997) summarized compelling data from several sources and concluded that even minimal hearing losses can cause problems with hearing, language, and learning, especially when the deficits are correlated with chronic middle ear disease.

   There are several other factors that preclude a simple, accurate description of the nature of hearing loss. For example, losses can affect one or both ears, be mild or profound, worse for some frequencies and better for others, congenital or acquired, temporary or permanent, facilitated with hearing aid use or not facilitated, and disabling to varying degrees. Care should be taken when describing a hearing loss, as simplistic statements can be misleading and not in a child's best interest.

What Are the Types and Common Causes of Hearing Loss in Children?

Hearing losses are generally identified as conductive, sensorineural, or mixed. Conductive losses refer to any obstruction in the conduction (transmission) of sound from the external ear to the inner ear. In such cases the inner ear is not damaged and is capable of transmitting information to the brain, providing the transmission link to the inner ear is functioning or can be bypassed. For example, the sound-conducting mechanism of the middle ear can be bypassed by directly stimulating the mastoid bone posterior to the external ear flap. The vibrations are thereby picked up by the fluid of the inner ear and processed without the assistance of the middle ear.

Certain congenital anomalies, childhood diseases, ear infections, and physical injuries to the ear can be responsible for a *conductive hearing loss*. Middle ear infection, or *otitis media*, is the largest cause of hearing loss in children. Frequently these infections affect the Eustachian tube function, causing middle ear air pressure to be less than adequate. This, along with the buildup of fluid in the cavity, often causes otitis media to be a very painful experience for a child. The common cold and various viruses are largely responsible for these infections. Decongestants, antihistamines, and antibiotics are frequently prescribed. If the problem persists, a myringotomy, or surgical incision of the eardrum, may be necessary to allow adequate pressure balance and fluid drainage from the middle ear. In addition to the discomfort associated with the infection, it is not atypical for a child to have a mild-to-moderate temporary conductive hearing loss. All in all, an acute condition of otitis media can be a disconcerting experience for a child. Classroom teachers need to be particularly supportive during these episodes.

Sensorineural hearing loss refers to disorders caused by problems in the cochlea, or the cochlear nerve. A pure sensory disorder has its origin in the cochlea, whereas a neural disorder stems primarily from pathology of the cochlear nerve. Sensorineural hearing losses are not "cured" by prescription drugs or by medical intervention of any sort. These losses are typically permanent and in some cases are progressive over time. Hearing losses of this nature are typically moderate to profound, and there are many potential causes. Genetic factors are responsible for many cases of congenital sensorineural hearing loss, but not all cases are congenital. Sometimes a congenital problem does not manifest itself until years after birth. Also, there are some congenital syndromes that include many other anomalies in addition to hearing loss.

Maternal viral infections can cause severe hearing loss and other problems in developing fetuses. Rubella (German measles) is a cyclical phenomenon, occurring in the past about every 7 years in the United States. However, a vaccine to prevent rubella has been developed, so we will be seeing many fewer cases of rubella-induced hearing loss. Other childhood viral diseases such as measles, mumps, chickenpox, and influenza also have the potential, albeit not great, to cause hearing loss. When a hearing deficit follows the mumps virus, it is ordinarily seen in one ear only. Cytomegalovirus, anoxia at birth, prematurity, birth trauma, Rh incompatibility, and meningitis are also correlated with hearing loss and brain damage.

While middle ear problems are the leading cause of hearing problems in children, the effects of aging and noise exposure are largely responsible for hearing loss in adults. Health professionals, however, are concerned about the impact of the "boom box" era on ears of persons under 18 (Alpiner & McCarthy, 1993). There is evidence that the prevalence of hearing loss is increasing for this age group because of the high levels of output from these sound sources (Chermak & Peters-

McCarthy, 1991). Hearing conservation programs are recommended for school children so they can be informed about the hazards of noise exposure.

Hearing loss is not always categorized as conductive or sensorineural. Children with permanent sensorineural losses are just as vulnerable to transient middle ear diseases as are those with normal hearing, and hearing loss in such children is *mixed*.

Two additional types of hearing loss are of special interest to the classroom teacher: functional and central. A functional loss is not a true hearing loss. That is, a child responds to auditory stimuli at high decibel levels when, in fact, true threshold levels are normal. In most cases the fake response is intentional, and there is usually some stress-related reason for it. Typically these problems are not serious, but they usually require professional intervention. Teachers need to be supportive of the child as the problem is being resolved. Less common is the situation in which a child is incapable of responding to auditory events in a normal manner, for various reasons, including emotional problems. School children with functional hearing disorders are rarely seen in regular classrooms.

Central auditory processing problems concern difficulty in the understanding of information received auditorially due to pathologies of the brainstem or hearing centers of the brain. Children with *central auditory processing problems* may have unimpaired peripheral hearing mechanisms but varying degrees of brain dysfunction. Accordingly, they may receive the sounds in the environment but show difficulty in fully interpreting the meaning of the sounds. They encounter their greatest processing difficulties when the listening environment is cluttered with background noise and speech. The problem generally manifests itself by characteristics of limited attention span, inability to follow verbal directions precisely, problems in mastering verbal materials, confusion with verbal communication, occasional aberrant behavior, and reading and writing problems. Parents and teachers often label these students as having behavior problems before they are diagnosed otherwise. It would not be incorrect, however, to apply the label of "special learning disorder."

Auditory attention deficits (ADD), typically not classified as hearing losses, can be considered auditory processing problems. A child who has difficulty focusing on a primary listening signal, maintaining attention to that signal, and shifting appropriately to another listening signal can be described as having an auditory attention deficit (Matkin, 1996). The child with this deficit, who also exhibits the behavioral tendencies just described, can logically be characterized as having an *attention deficit hyperactivity disorder* (ADHD). Research suggests that these are biologically based disorders and that children with these problems are typically distractible, impulsive, and often hyperactive (Widmeyer Group, 1994).

The existence of central auditory processing and auditory attention problems is not easily determined. The educational psychologist, learning disorders specialist, audiologist, speech-language pathologist, and neurologist all may have a significant role in the diagnostic and intervention process. The psychologist and learning disorders specialist can determine whether the problem is a specific learning disorder or a generalized learning problem. The audiologist can identify the type and magnitude of auditory dysfunction and provide evidence in support of the presence or absence of an auditory processing problem. The speech-language pathologist can evaluate the impact the disorder has on receptive and expressive language performance and provide guidance for an appropriate intervention program. Finally, the neurologist can verify the presence of a brain dysfunction and, when appropriate, provide medical intervention.

The classroom teacher may wish to initiate the evaluation process with any of these specialists. Should such a disorder be identified, the efforts of all the specialists, as well as the assistance of the classroom teacher and the child's family members, may be crucial to the success of the remediation.

What Are the Classifications of Hearing Loss?

Most adults have observed the significant communication problems of deaf children. Deaf children generally exhibit hearing losses in excess of 90 decibels, have little or no functional hearing, and often have limited capability for oral speech. Deaf children are usually diagnosed as such before school age because their receptive and expressive communication problems are more readily observed. There are substantially more children, however, with slight hearing losses whose hearing difficulties are noted only under poor acoustic conditions. Excessively reverberant classrooms and seating at a distance create listening problems for these students. Their speech, however, is rarely affected. Diagnosis of the child with a slight hearing loss is often elusive because symptomatology is not as apparent. Before diagnosis these students typically are described as inattentive, restless, daydreamers, and as having difficulty in following directions.

Deafness and *minimal hearing loss* are terms signifying the extremes of a classification system of hearing impairment. Each category of hearing loss presents a unique constellation of diagnostic, educational, and emotional adjustment considerations. Although varying in numbers, all classifications are encountered in the schools (see Table 6-1).

Hearing impaired is a generic term for all types and degrees of hearing loss. Often, modifiers such as "mild," "moderate," "severe," and "profound" are included to denote the degree of hearing impairment (e.g., "moderately hearing impaired").

The *hard of hearing* category includes all degrees of hearing loss except the classification of deaf. Children in this group have hearing losses ranging from 15 to 75 dB. Their speech and language skills are developed primarily through the use of *hearing*, although lipreading and hearing aids are often very important as well.

TABLE 6-1   Classes of Hearing Handicap

dB	Degree of Handicap and Ability to Hear Speech
15–25	*Minimal handicap.* Difficulty with faint speech.
26–45	*Mild.* Frequent difficulty with normal speech.
46–65	*Moderate.* Frequent difficulty with loud speech.
66–85	*Severe.* Speech may be heard with amplification.
86–100	*Profound.* May not use hearing for communication.

Deaf children, those with severe hearing deficits, do not rely on hearing for learning or for the development of language and speech. They are highly dependent upon visual systems such as lipreading, fingerspelling, and sign language. Most deaf children have some residual hearing, usually in the very low frequencies.

What Is the Prevalence of Hearing Loss in Children?

It has been reported that there are 16 to 30 times more hard of hearing children than deaf children, and it is commonly accepted that the prevalence of deaf persons is about 1 per 1,000 of the general population (Ross, Brackett, & Maxon, 1991). It would appear, therefore, that the number of children with educationally significant hearing losses falls somewhere between 16 and 30 per 1000. Also, it can be concluded that the incidence of deafness is relatively rare compared to the number of those identified as hard of hearing.

Case History

Brian

Brian, a second-grader and an excellent student, had just had a week-long illness that included severe earaches and fever. When the pain and fever subsided, his parents concluded that the illness had run its course. Brian had indicated his desire to return to school and had said that he felt good.

During Brian's second day back at school, the teacher gave a spelling test, on which he did poorly. During oral reading sessions with his group, Brian had difficulty following the class recitations. He appeared to be inattentive, followed instructions inconsistently, and eventually provoked the teacher to admonish him for his lack of attention. These characteristics typified his behavior for the next few days. Brian cried easily and began to withdraw from classroom involvement. The teacher began to be concerned, as Brian was generally a very good student. He did not appear ill, and the teacher was at a loss to explain his atypical behavior. The single, new mannerism she did note was that he tugged at his earlobes often. The teacher decided to have a discussion with him to find out if there was a problem she could help resolve. Brian told the teacher he felt well but that he had trouble listening and understanding. In addition, he said that his ears felt as if they were full of water, but they did not hurt.

The teacher contacted the speech-language pathologist to have his hearing tested. Test results showed that Brian had sustained a significant conductive hearing loss in both ears. He was referred to a physician and was given medication to reduce the fluid levels in his middle ears. Within a short period of time his hearing had returned to normal and so had his behavior and schoolwork. The teacher's early awareness and willingness to help a youngster whose behavior signaled a problem may have prevented a chronic middle ear problem from developing.

Summary

Causes of Hearing Loss

- Physical anomalies of the ear
- Childhood diseases
- Ear infections (especially otitis media)
- Eustachian tube dysfunction
- Common colds
- Certain antibiotics and drugs
- Genetic factors
- Maternal viral infections (especially rubella)
- Anoxia at birth
- Birth trauma
- Blows to the head and acoustic trauma
- Rh incompatibility
- Brain damage

Some Important Points to Remember

- A significant hearing loss can cause serious language, voice, and articulation problems.
- The magnitude of hearing loss is expressed in decibels.
- The more decibels of hearing loss, the poorer one can hear.
- Hearing loss for one or two frequencies does not cause a problem with hearing.
- The interpretation of what is heard is completed by the brain.
- The meaning that is attached to the sounds in the environment is learned.
- Pure tones and speech signals are used in routine audiometry.
- Hearing loss is plotted on an audiogram.
- An "X" signals left ear responses; "O" signals right ear responses.
- The number of decibels below the zero line on the audiogram indicates the decibels of hearing loss.
- Hearing loss in only one ear usually does not mean a child will have a school learning problem.
- Children acquiring hearing losses before the development of language usually present more serious problems.
- Conductive hearing losses, which are often treatable, are related to obstructions in the transmission of sound to the inner ear.
- Sensorineural hearing losses usually are not reversible.
- Central auditory processing problems are special cases of specific learning disorders.
- Children with central auditory processing problems often have normal hearing sensitivity.
- Diagnosis of the child with a slight hearing loss is often elusive, as symptomology is not apparent.

- The term *hearing impaired* is a generic term referring to all types and degrees of hearing loss.
- *Hard of hearing* children usually rely on residual hearing and lipreading for learning.
- *Deaf* children often rely on fingerspelling, sign language, and lipreading for learning and communication.
- There are about 16–30 times more hard of hearing than deaf children.
- It is commonly reported that one in every thousand persons is deaf.

Self-Test

Multiple Choice:

1. The rate of vibrations in a sound is expressed in:

   A. Decibels
   B. Hertz
   C. intensity
   D. dB
   E. loudness

2. Speech is an excellent example of:

   A. a pure tone
   B. a single vibratory rate
   C. a complex sound
   D. a single sound pressure wave

3. The meaning associated with a sound is processed in:

   A. the middle ear
   B. the brain
   C. the inner ear
   D. the cochlea

4. The frequency of a tone corresponds to its:

   A. loudness
   B. intensity
   C. pitch
   D. decibel level

5. The important frequency range for hearing speech is between:

   A. 300 and 4,000 Hz
   B. 5,000 and 10,000 Hz
   C. 12,000 and 18,000 Hz
   D. 300 and 4,000 dB
   E. 12,000 and 18,000 dB

6. Hearing with two ears is most important for recognizing the:

   A. frequency of the sound
   B. intensity of the sound
   C. complexity of the sound
   D. location of the sound
   E. pitch of the sound

7. Normal atmospheric pressure within the middle ear is achieved through the:

   A. cochlea
   B. stapes
   C. both A and B
   D. Eustachian tube
   E. ossicles

8. Meaning that is attached to the sound of our environment is:

   A. learned
   B. innate
   C. acquired only after 24 months of age
   D. all of the above
   E. none of the above

9. With normal hearing, children typically develop mature articulation of speech sounds between the ages of:

   A. 6 and 8
   B. 2 and 3
   C. 10 and 12
   D. none of the above

10. While testing an individual's hearing, sensitivity threshold levels for various frequencies are plotted on a form called a(n):

    A. scatterplot
    B. audiogram
    C. audiometer
    D. decibel graph
    E. tone profile

11. The largest cause of hearing loss in children is:

    A. mumps
    B. rubella
    C. otitis media
    D. cytomegalovirus
    E. none of the above

12. Sensorineural hearing losses are:

    A. typically permanent
    B. not readily "cured" by prescription drugs

     C.   sometimes progressive over time

     D.   all of the above

     E.   none of the above

13. Children with central auditory processing problems:

     A.   typically receive sound in the environment, but show difficulty in fully interpreting the meaning of the sound

     B.   often have most difficulty when the listening environment is cluttered with background noise

     C.   have conductive hearing loss problems

     D.   both A and B

14. The term *hearing impairment* is:

     A.   used synonymously with *deafness* only

     B.   used synonymously with *hard of hearing* only

     C.   a generic term relating to all types and degrees of hearing loss

     D.   none of the above

15. Deaf children:

     A.   rely on hearing for the development of speech and language

     B.   typically have substantial hearing ability

     C.   are highly dependent upon visual systems such as sign language and lipreading

     D.   can never develop oral speech

References

Alpiner, G., & McCarthy, P. (1993). *Rehabilitative audiology: Children and adults*. Baltimore, MD: Williams & Wilkins.

Chermak, G., & Peters-McCarthy, E. (1991). The effectiveness of an educational hearing conservation program for elementary school children. *Language, Speech, and Hearing Services in Schools, 22*, 308–312.

Martin, F. (1997). *Introduction to audiology*. Boston: Allyn & Bacon.

Martin, F., & Clark, J. (1996). *Hearing care for children*. Boston: Allyn & Bacon.

Matkin, N. (1996). The potential benefits of amplification for young children with normal hearing.

In *Amplification for children with auditory deficits*. Nashville, TN: Bill Wilkerson Center Press.

Roberts, J., Wallace, I., & Henderson, F. (Eds.). (1997). *Otitis media in young children*. Baltimore, MD: Brookes.

Ross, M., Brackett, D., & Maxon, A. (1991). *Assessment and management of mainstreamed hearing-impaired children*. Austin, TX: Pro-Ed.

Widmeyer Group. (1994). *Attention deficit disorder: Beyond the myths*. Part of contract #HS9201700. Washington, DC: Office of Special Education Programs, Office of Special Education and Rehabilitative Services, U.S. Dept. of Education.

Chapter *7*

School Children with Hearing Impairments

This chapter addresses the management of children with hearing impairments under the provisions of federal legislation, the Individuals with Disabilities Education Act (IDEA) of 1997. Under the aegis of this law, appropriate services for hearing-impaired children from birth to 21 years of age are ensured. As a result, detection and management of hearing loss can occur at a very early age for hearing-impaired children and increase their potential for educational achievement and personal adjustment. Early intervention also takes advantage of the formative language development period between 6 months and 4 years of age.

How Are Hearing Losses Detected?

What Screening Procedures Are Available?

Infants and toddlers cannot reliably indicate whether they can hear a sound or not. Accordingly, various hearing screening procedures have been developed that do not require their cooperation. A widely used technique called *otoacoustic emissions* (OAE) is quick and efficient and now routine in testing newborns. A miniature microphone and a small earphone are placed in the ear canal. Sounds are presented through the microphone and the normal ear will respond back with an echo of the sound. Another procedure commonly used with infants, toddlers, and young children is called the auditory brainstem response (ABR). In this method, sounds are presented to the child's ears through earphones while the child sleeps. Responses are recorded from electrophysiological readings transmitted via electrodes coupled to the head. Other techniques exploit a child's developing ability to localize sound, a skill that emerges around 3 to 5 months of age. In this method the child is conditioned to look in the direction of sounds emanating from strategically placed loudspeakers. For example, a tone is generated from a speaker to the right of a child's head position. Immediately following the tone burst a captivating visual reinforcer, such as toy dancing clowns, is activated in the immediate vicinity of the speaker. If the child hears the stimulus, he or she should look in the direction of the speaker. It is assumed the child wants to see the dancing clowns again so that when other sounds are generated there is motivation to look in the direction of the sound source and thereby signal the sound was heard.

Hearing screening programs for children in grades K through 12 are fairly routine. The screening procedures used usually include a pure tone audiometric screening to determine a child's ability to detect certain frequencies at a preset decibel level. This is not a threshold test but is a "pass" or "fail" technique for each frequency used. In addition, screening tympanometry is ordinarily employed. This test is an indirect measure of the integrity of the middle ear. The procedure evaluates how readily the eardrum accepts energy as small changes in air pressure are induced in the external ear canal. The technique measures not only the mobility of the eardrum but also the function of the Eustachian tube. As a result, slight conductive hearing losses can be identified, which might otherwise be missed by pure tone screening.

If a child performs poorly on either of these tests, a followup test with an audiologist is scheduled. Conventional pure tone audiometry, tympanometry, and other tests are employed as needed. Should a child exhibit a hearing loss of any type, a referral to an appropriate physician is usually made.

Can a Teacher Identify Hearing Loss in Students?

There is no sure way to recognize hearing loss in children simply by observing their behavior. Nonetheless, teachers often do suspect hearing loss in students and make the appropriate referrals to confirm or reject their suspicions. Deficient hearing may be suspected if a child (1) asks for spoken messages to be repeated, (2) frequently misunderstands what has been said, (3) cups ears or tilts head in the direction of a sound, (4) shows facial expressions suggesting inattention to what is being said, (5) speaks louder than the situation dictates, or (6) withdraws from situations requiring listening.

Teachers are advised to pay particular attention to students who have a history of ear disease or who often complain of ear discomfort. It should be emphasized that the only reliable method for identifying hearing loss is audiometric testing by a trained person.

What Types of Speech and Language Problems Do Children with Hearing Impairments Have?

In general, children *born* with hearing loss (referred to as prelingual or congenital losses) have significantly greater speech and language problems than children who incur losses after speech has developed (postlingual losses). Typically children with congenital hearing loss are less intelligible and have less potential for learning articulate speech because they have not had the opportunity to hear normal speech.

Children with hearing impairments essentially produce speech as they hear it. They tend to omit consonants, especially voiceless consonants, that occur at the ends of words. Final consonants are ordinarily unstressed, inherently weaker in speech power than when produced in other parts of words, and are not easily heard by the hearing-impaired child. In addition, they often prolong and nasalize the preceding vowels. Consonants using tongue tip placements such as *t* tend to be omitted regardless of relative position within words. Another common problem concerns voicing certain speech sounds that should not be voiced.

Numerous factors, including intelligence, socioeconomic class, parental involvement, age of onset of hearing loss, and effective use of amplification, affect language competence more than speech articulation proficiency. There are some trends, however, that are worth noting. Hard of hearing children consistently show a 2- to 3-year lag in vocabulary development, while deaf children show a significantly wider gap (Ross, Brackett, & Maxon, 1991). Children with hearing impairments encounter the most difficulty with idiomatic expressions, colloquialisms, and other uses of words beyond their dictionary meanings and are often deficient in use of synonyms. Syntactical constructions pose problems and, again, there is a correlation with degree of hearing loss; children with mild losses often perform like children with normal hearing, whereas children with severe losses show numerous problems with complex grammatical constructions.

How Do Children with Hearing Impairments Learn Language and Speech?

Hard of Hearing Children

Hard of hearing children, those who can understand speech if it is loud enough, learn their language and speech skills much like normal hearing children, primarily through the sense of hearing. The IEP team, usually led by the speech-language pathologist, guides the assistance, which may include auditory training, using a personal hearing aid, language stimulation, lipreading, and speech training. Parents have the major role during the early years, and as the child approaches formal schooling there is more intensive involvement by the speech-language clinician. In general, children with more significant degrees of hearing loss require more intensive intervention and over a longer time span, often for several years.

A major goal for the child classified as hard of hearing is to learn spoken language. The teaching methodologies, which do not vary significantly, have been labeled *auditory-global* and *auditory-visual-oral*. Both are relatively effective if efficiently employed. Each stresses practice in listening using a properly fitting hearing aid, language stimulation, and training in the production of speech sounds.

The auditory-global method relies more heavily on the development of residual hearing, the area of hearing that can be enhanced by an appropriate hearing aid. The method is also referred to as *auditory-oral, aural-oral, auditory,* or *acoupedics.* Because hearing and listening are stressed, it is considered unisensory. The development of oralism is treated through hearing only. The professionals who use this method emphasize that hearing-impaired children grow up in a hearing world and therefore must survive the forces of a hearing society. Accordingly, teaching should focus on listening, with language and speech development as logical products. They note that humans are neurologically predisposed to learn language and that language is learned ideally by hearing it. While the popular view is that the method is highly appropriate for children who have mild to moderate hearing losses, many proponents insist that it is the treatment of choice, regardless of degree of hearing loss.

The *auditory-visual-oral* method is similar to the auditory-global approach. Hearing, listening, and speech are stressed. The difference is in the incorporation of a multisensory approach using lipreading (also referred to as speech-reading) along with listening, and the discretionary use of tactile stimulation. Although lipreading may not be taught systematically, children are encouraged to use all the information available by watching lip, tongue, and jaw movements that coincide with the sounds of speech that are produced. Advocates point out that the speech sounds that are not heard by persons with high-frequency hearing losses are often the sounds that are more lipreadable. As a result, lipreading supplements hearing and improves one's ability to more fully understand the spoken message. Tactile stimulation can also supplement lipreading ability for those with severe losses. Transducers that change acoustic stimuli to vibratory information can be worn as stimulators on the wrists, fingertips, or back.

Another method, loosely related to the methods discussed, is *cued speech* (Cornett, 1967). Eight hand configurations and four hand placements used in positions around the speech articulators provide cues about certain speech sounds that are otherwise visually obscure. The availability of this information also promotes teaching children with hearing impairments the production of speech sounds. The cueing is totally dependent upon speech and is meaningless out of context. Cued speech is not a sign language but rather a supplement to lipreading and an aid to teaching speech.

For hard of hearing children with more severe degrees of hearing loss, the *Rochester method* is a pedagogical option. Named after the school for deaf children in Rochester, New York, the approach uses hearing, lipreading, and fingerspelling simultaneously. As with cued speech, the method purports to provide missing information not accessed through hearing or lipreading, using hand configurations that represent each of the 26 letters of the alphabet. Speakers fingerspell words as they are spoken. The Rochester method is also referred to as visible speech.

The methodologies that emphasize reliance on hearing and speech share the basic goal of providing means for children with hearing impairments to be integrated and functional in the hearing world. Early identification, early use of amplification, intensive auditory training and speech training, commitment of family, and special educational intervention strategies are important to their success.

There is little controversy about the appropriateness of these methods for children classified as hard of hearing.

Deaf Children

There has been controversy about the efficacy of the auditory-oral methods for deaf children, those children with audiograms showing hearing losses in excess of 80 to 90 dBs. For years many older deaf persons and professionals have been concerned about the lack of success in communicating and teaching language to deaf children through speech and hearing. They have urged the educational establishment to accept *manual* approaches (sign language) over *oral* approaches (speech and lipreading). The oralists fear the use of sign language will impede oral language and speech acquisition, while manualists claim the oral approach is often impractical and too difficult for most deaf persons to master.

The manualists also contend that forcing deaf children to communicate only through speech and lipreading denies them full and successful communication through sign language, an efficient communication mode for them. Data show that deaf adults overwhelmingly prefer sign language and that many vigorously promote the teaching of signs to deaf children as the primary form of language expression and learning (Moores, 1987). The opposing view is that our "brains are wired" to learn language by hearing it and that there is no adequate substitute for hearing and speech. These proponents hold that most deaf children are capable of hearing some speech components with properly fitting hearing aids and that the challenge is to maximize their auditory capabilities.

A compromise approach, *total communication*, is the simultaneous use of sign language and auditory-oral methods. The total communication philosophy is touted as highly appropriate for deaf children who acquire deafness before the acquisition of language. It requires that each deaf child be provided aural, oral, and manual modes of communication in any combination that will best facilitate learning, effective communication, and personal adjustment. The philosophy incorporates the view that each deaf child deserves a communication method that is individualized and considers degree of hearing loss, family support, professional facilities and expertise, social and intellectual abilities, and any other variable that significantly influences the potential for success. Today this concept is widely embraced as an appropriate framework for the education of children with hearing impairments.

Oralists complain, however, that any incorporation of American Sign Language fosters confusion among deaf children about the nature of English and how to read and write it. To accommodate this concern, some educators have devised modifications to traditional sign language so that it will more closely correlate with spoken English. The following sections compare the merits of American Sign Language and the use of sign codes.

American Sign Language, also known as *AMESLAN* or *ASL*, is a bona fide language in its own right. It has its own vocabulary structure, grammar, and idiomatic form. It is a nonoral language and therefore has inherent value to a deaf person. In this sense, ASL is often referred to as the native language of deaf persons.

When ASL is taught to deaf children at a very early age, it has been shown that these children learn sign language at about the same rate normal hearing children acquire spoken language (Moores, 1987). Accordingly, effective communication skills are not unduly denied the deaf child during the early preschool years. But a deaf child who does not know English will not be able to read and write English. For this reason many educators acknowledge the importance of compromising the use of ASL for another system of signs that more closely correlates with English vocabulary and grammar. This has led to the development of various sign codes.

Sign codes do not qualify as separate languages, although they are often loosely referred to as sign language systems. While signs are used, the grammar and vocabulary are essentially English. These systems are designed to enhance the educational success of deaf children by providing an opportunity to learn English language skills. As a result, proficiency in the reading and writing of English is more likely to result.

Pidgin is a true compromise between ASL and English. The English grammar is intact, the vocabulary is ASL, and English is spoken with the simultaneous use of signs that carry important meaning. A deaf child who does not know English, however, cannot lipread the words or parts of words that are not signed. *Signed English* is similar to Pidgin in that the signed vocabulary is drawn from ASL and the word order follows English grammar. But an exact representation of the English language is only possible by using extensive fingerspelling and providing special signs for prefixes, suffixes, plural endings, and articles such as "the," "a," and "an." Users of Signed English appear to adapt to ASL readily, and ASL users find Signed English translatable, albeit cumbersome and redundant.

Hearing Aids and Assistive Listening Devices

Hearing aids and assistive listening devices help hearing-impaired individuals receive and interpret information presented auditorially. *Hearing aids* are electronic devices that make sounds louder but do not provide corrective hearing the same way eyeglasses might correct visual acuity problems. If residual hearing does not exist for certain frequencies, a hearing aid will not provide it. Where residual hearing exists, a hearing aid will make sounds louder in that range of hearing. *Assistive listening devices* (Figure 7-1) are systems engineered for specific listening conditions such as theaters, concert halls, churches, civic centers, various sports arenas, and for special use in the home. In most situations, ear phones or ear inserts are electronically connected to an amplifying system designed for the environment. Typically these systems rely on a direct connection to the intended sound source while blocking out intervening sounds in the environment. As a result, persons with hearing impairments can circumvent the noise distractions that would accompany listening through a personal hearing aid. Other types of assistive listening devices serve as warning, alerting, or wake-up systems. A vibrator placed under a pillow is an example of a wake-up device. A flashing lightbulb situated over a door might indicate the doorbell is ringing. A large flashing red light can be designed to signal a fire alarm has been triggered. There are

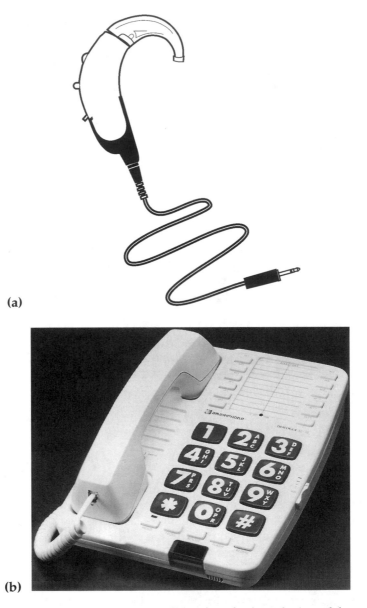

(a)

(b)

FIGURE 7-1   **Examples of assistive listening devices designed for use by individuals with hearing impairments: (a) a hearing aid that is coupled by a direct connection with a sound source to block intervening sounds in the environment; (b) a telephone with special controls to regulate the degree of amplified sound required by the user; (c) an FM transmitter with headset and receiver, which can also circumvent the intervention of environmental sounds; (d) a transmitter and combination receiver-headset that uses infrared technology. Photographs courtesy of Siemens Hearing Instruments, Inc.**

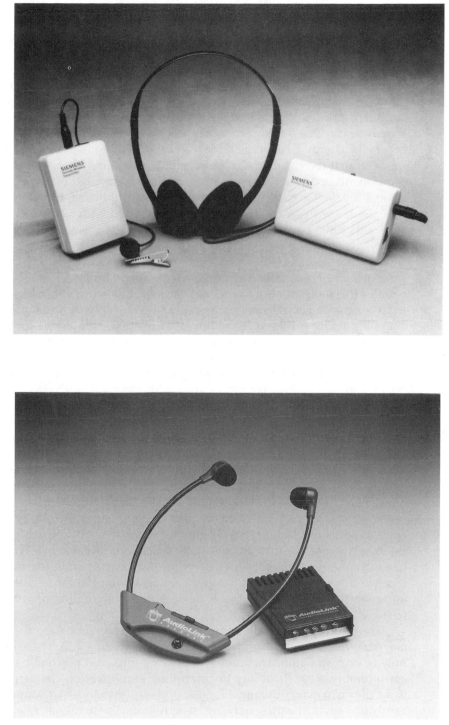

(c)

(d)

numerous such devices that help people with hearing impairments function more efficiently in a world filled with auditory signals and alerts. The audiologist or speech-language pathologist can help families secure appropriate devices for a child with a hearing loss.

There has been significant progress in improving the fidelity and cosmetic appearance of personal hearing aids. Regardless of size or appearance, all have three basic components. All electronic hearing aids have a *microphone* that picks up auditory signals in the environment. The microphone also changes the nature of the signals to electrical energy and channels the signals to an amplifier. The *amplifier* boosts the energy level of the signals and routes them to a *receiver* (miniature loud-speaker) that reconverts the electrical signals back to auditory signals. These basic components are powered by a battery and supplemented by various switches that change tonal characteristics, turn the aid on or off, or manipulate volume control.

Persons with severe hearing loss may be fitted with a *body hearing aid* because such aids have larger compartments to hold bigger batteries, resulting in more power for amplification. Body aids are usually worn in a pocket on a blouse or shirt or in a special holder worn under the outer garments. The metal or plastic compartment houses the microphone, amplifier, and batteries. An electrical cord couples the compartment to the receiver, which is worn at ear level and connects to an ear mold. The ear mold is specially fitted for the ear and not only provides a coupling device for the receiver but also directs the amplified sound into the ear canal. Because the body aid separates the microphone from the speaker by several inches, there is less likelihood that a problem with feedback will occur.

Another style of hearing aid is the *behind-the-ear* (or over-the-ear) aid. All components are at ear level, and while these aids can equal the power of the body aid, the proximity of the microphone and receiver can cause a feedback problem when extra volume is needed. The plastic compartment is worn directly behind the ear or in eyeglass stems and houses the microphone, receiver, and battery. The amplified sound is routed through a plastic tube from the compartment to an ear mold. Because these aids have good fidelity and are capable of providing high levels of amplification, they are frequently recommended for children with significant losses.

A newer style of ear-level amplification is the *in-the-ear* hearing aid. The entire hearing aid is contained within the plastic shell of an ear mold. There are no connecting wires or plastic tubes. Technology now makes it possible to miniaturize these aids so that the instrument can fit entirely in the ear canal. These are referred to as *canal* aids. With all types of in-the-ear hearing aids the microphone and receiver are very close in proximity, causing a potential for feedback. As a result, audiologists tend to prefer larger devices for young children with severe losses. (See Figure 7-2.)

The development of the computer microchip has promoted the engineering of *programmable hearing aids* and *digital hearing aids* (Figure 7-2). These instruments are now worn by a significant number of hearing-impaired persons, as they give users considerably more flexibility in controlling amplification characteristics. Specifically, they can quiet unwanted loud sounds and enhance soft sounds, thus significantly improving hearing in noisy backgrounds, the nemesis of hearing aid users.

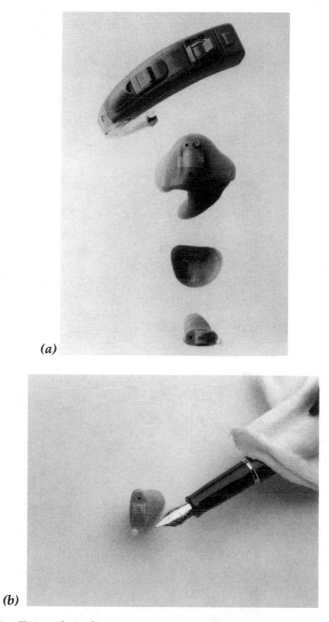

(a)

(b)

FIGURE 7-2   **Examples of personal hearing aids. All aids shown represent current technology and are digital or programmable in design. (a) from top to bottom, an over-the-ear aid; an all in-the-ear aid, a canal aid, and a small canal aid worn totally in the ear canal, (b) the small canal aid compared to the tip of a fountain pen; (c) an over-the-ear aid fitted to a user's ear; (d) an in-the-ear aid fitted to a user's ear. (Photographs courtesy of Siemens Hearing Instruments, Inc.)**

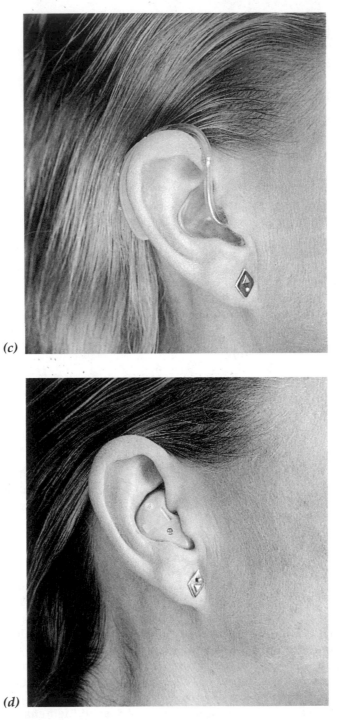

(c)

(d)

FIGURE 7-2   *Continued*

In addition, the user can adjust the instrument to compensate for varying listening situations—restaurants, churches, theaters, et cetera. The major drawback is the relatively high price of these devices.

The reader should be aware that personal hearing aids are a vital component of auditory habilitation for hard of hearing children. They provide the potential to bring the sounds of speech into the range of hearing, sounds that otherwise would not be readily heard. Also, a student's personal adjustment and success in school can be enhanced with an optimally fitted instrument. Auditory training is designed to maximize the potential of amplified sound. Deaf children, however, do not benefit as much from amplified sound because the severity of hearing loss prohibits the reception of meaningful speech. Some deaf children, however, enjoy amplified sound even though it is little more than fragmentary information about speech, the fact someone is speaking, and information about the tempo and rhythm of the speech. Others rely on their hearing aids to provide clues about alerting signals in the environment, signals correlated with a car horn, a bell, or a siren. And still others consider a hearing aid more of a nuisance than a benefit.

Modern technology has facilitated the development of *cochlear implants*, and these devices offer new opportunities for certain individuals. A cochlear implant, however, is not a hearing aid. An implant does not amplify sound and send it into the ear canal. As the name implies, there is an implantation of a device that includes a receiver and a wire electrode in the mastoid process behind the pinna. In addition, there are external parts—a microphone near the ear, a signal processor worn like a body aid, and a stimulator coupled to the implanted device. Unlike hearing aids per se, the cochlear implant changes sound into electrical current that is sent directly to the inner ear. Thus, the ear is not truly stimulated with sound, but rather with electrical energy. Accordingly, what is perceived is quite different from what one hears by the way of acoustical energy.

Cochlear implants are not for everyone with a hearing loss. To date, relatively few are considered good candidates. Clearly those who have known normal hearing and have acquired profound losses are better candidates than those with congenital deafness. Also, implant recipients' accounts of the quality of the information they receive vary. Some perceive the basic components of speech signals better than others. In some cases, only information about the rhythm, duration, and loudness of speech is received. A considerable number claim their lipreading skills are significantly enhanced. Regardless, researchers are optimistic about the future of cochlear implants, especially for children with profound losses.

It is important to remember that people with hearing impairments speak their language very much the way they hear it. With appropriate intervention and by wearing a properly fitting hearing aid, most hard of hearing individuals can learn to understand English through hearing and lipreading and can learn to speak effectively. Because deaf children hear very little speech and hearing aids cannot provide hearing where residual hearing does not exist, learning through hearing can be a tortuous ordeal for them. Intervention strategies that focus mainly on visual communication skills such as fingerspelling, sign codes, and sign language offer a better potential for this group.

What Special School Programs Are Provided for Children with Hearing Impairments?

Because learning is dependent upon language skills, and because hard of hearing children are communicatively deficient, guidance from the speech-language pathologist is often critical to the success of these students. This coordinating role does not presume that the work of this professional is more important than that of the classroom teacher. In the final analysis the classroom teacher has the overall responsibility for learning by all students in the classroom.

Many children with significant hearing impairments are not mainstreamed into regular classroom settings. Special classrooms instructed by specially trained teachers of the deaf are often provided for these students so that their unique learning needs can be met. (Not all children assigned to special classes for the deaf are categorized as deaf.) These classes are usually very small (six to eight students) and rely heavily on visual aids for instruction. It is not uncommon for sign language to be the primary means of communication. Special language instruction is often provided by a speech-language pathologist.

If a child is mainstreamed into a regular classroom and is dependent upon sign language for communication, it is usually necessary to provide an interpreter for the deaf to assist the classroom teacher. Programs for mainstreamed hard of hearing children usually include substantial assistance by a speech-language pathologist. For those children with moderate (45 to 65 dB) and severe (65 to 85 dB) hearing losses a hearing resource teacher is often provided. These professionals provide tutoring in support of the regular classroom curriculum, whereas speech-language pathologists focus on listening, language, and speech instruction.

What Is the Role of the Classroom Teacher?

The importance of the classroom teacher in the overall education of a hearing-impaired child must not be underestimated. Not all teachers, however, have the disposition or patience to meet the challenge and fulfill the time-consuming responsibilities associated with efficient management of these children. There are numerous special considerations that are vital to the success of the regular classroom experience for the child with a hearing impairment. A discussion of these considerations follows.

The teacher has a role in ensuring that a hearing-impaired child has an optimal hearing and listening environment in the classroom. This means that there should be minimal distance between the teacher and the child. As listening becomes more difficult, the child will rely more on visual information. Therefore, the arrangement should also consider good lighting, so the child can take advantage of important visual clues such as lipreading. The teacher is urged to keep classroom noise to a minimum, as the effective use of a hearing aid requires a relatively quiet listening environment. Too many classrooms have been found to be excessively noisy and not appropriate for the learning of a hearing-impaired child using amplification (Ross, Brackett, & Maxon, 1991; Crandell & Smaldino, 1996).

The teacher should frequently check to see if the hearing aid is being worn and is functioning adequately. There are so many different types of hearing aids that it is difficult to know how to check their functioning, so close communication with the speech-language pathologist or audiologist in this regard will be of significant value to the teacher.

The teacher has a critical role in the emotional well-being and development of a hearing-impaired child. The classroom and playground can be the location of devastating experiences or they can foster healthy growth and development. It is to everyone's advantage for the teacher to be open about a child's hearing disability. When the appropriate opportunities surface, the teacher should explain hearing loss to the other children and encourage them to help the child with a disability learn and enjoy a rewarding school experience.

The classroom teacher has a responsibility to promote efficient, routine communication with all persons working toward the educational betterment of a child. This includes parents, special teachers, school testing personnel, speech-language pathologists, audiologists, counselors, and school administrators. Information sharing is critical and the teacher often is in the best position to facilitate it.

It is a daily challenge to foster the optimal mainstreaming of a child with a hearing impairment. It may seem expedient to treat the child like a special observer of the classroom, without expecting or encouraging participation or planning the integration of the child's needs, talents, and learning experiences. However, the teacher should explore feasible tactics that truly provide a mainstreamed environment.

The teacher should be fully informed about a hearing-impaired child's performance standards and potential. Little realistic planning or teaching can ensue without this information. The most critical information concerns language performance. The teacher must know the level and limits of the child's receptive vocabulary and syntax so that effective communication can take place.

The teacher needs to set realistic educational goals. Many mainstreamed hearing-impaired students cannot achieve the same goals as their hearing peers. There is a correlation between degree of hearing loss and language-based achievement. To expect or demand unrealistic performance in the classroom can be a source of frustration for the teacher, student, and parents.

Teachers should keep these points in mind when working with a child with a hearing impairment:

- Face the child during all oral communication.
- Do not exaggerate the pronunciation of words, as this will deter, not facilitate, understanding.
- Frequently check with the child to make sure he or she is comprehending.
- Use appropriate visual teaching aids whenever practical.
- Encourage the child to ask questions whenever necessary.
- Assign a hearing peer to be a "buddy" during extracurricular activities. This should assist the hearing-impaired child to be an active participant as well as provide a special helper to support effective communication.
- Learn to "read" the child's facial expressions in order to have feedback about his or her understanding or the material presented.

The Internet provides several excellent resources for teachers and parents concerning the education and well-being of children with hearing impairments. The Audiology Department of the Boys Town National Research Hospital in Omaha, Nebraska, has an excellent research and clinical facility and public information service. Information on numerous topics can be found at *www.boystown.org*. Three excellent resources on the effects of noise on school-age children and the components of effective hearing conservation programs in the schools are *www.hearing-education.com*, *www.hearingconservation.org*, and *www.lbb.org*. Information from the National Information Center for Children and Youth with Disabilities can be accessed at *www.nichcy.org*. The resources of Gallaudet University can be accessed via *www.gallaudet.edu*.

If the reader is in need of a better understanding of the basic tenets and legal ramifications of federal legislation concerning the management of children with hearing impairments, a well-organized and lucidly presented reference manual is *IDEA Advocacy for Children Who Are Deaf or Hard of Hearing* by B. P. Tucker, J.D. (see References).

Case Histories

Donald

Donald is a 6-year-old student at a public elementary school. At the age of 4 he had a viral illness that resulted in a bilateral sensorineural hearing loss of moderate degree with a greater loss for the high frequencies. Before his sickness he was considered to have high verbal skills and had no difficulty using oral language. Donald has been fitted with hearing aids for both ears and he wears them consistently. Test results using the aids show that he has normal hearing sensitivity for all frequencies except for 2000 Hertz and above. In this region his aided audiogram shows a consistent loss of about 30 dB. This causes him to miss many of the voiceless consonants when in noisy listening conditions, especially in the classroom.

Donald is placed in a regular classroom and individually sees a speech-language pathologist three times a week. The speech-language pathologist's objectives include training to help Donald retain articulatory proficiency for those speech sounds that are not clearly heard. In addition, he is receiving auditory training so he can use his hearing aid maximally. The clinician provides coping strategies for him as he meets the challenges of auditory failure during his day-to-day experiences. The clinician also confers with the classroom teacher frequently so that the classroom environment does not become an educationally restrictive setting for Donald. Topics such as preferential seating options, noise reduction in the classroom, and the use of special academic resources like visual aids are discussed. The teacher is also apprised of the goals and objectives of the special speech sessions so expectancies for carryover into the classroom can be monitored.

The key members of the IEP team are the parents, teacher, and the speech-language pathologist. As Donald represents a case that is not severe or complicated, there is high expectancy that he will develop educationally, and communicatively, at the same pace as his normal hearing peers. This, however, is contingent upon continued participation and cooperation of all the team members. Should family support and professional services not be available, there is the potential for deviant speech patterns to emerge and some minor language delay to occur. This, in turn, would have a negative impact on academic achievement. The IEP team, however, is optimistic about Donald's potential for academic success.

Theresa

Theresa, a 10-year-old Hispanic deaf child who is being reared by her maternal grandmother, now resides in a residential school for the deaf in her state. Her family lives in a small, English-speaking community in the South and has very limited financial resources. Although the Spanish language is spoken in a home that shelters six individual family members, the other children have some English speaking skills that were learned in the local public school.

Theresa was not diagnosed as deaf until she was 3 years old. Shortly thereafter the family was given special assistance by the school through the services of a speech-language pathologist. There was an early attempt to focus on oral language development, but the conflict between using Spanish and English proved to be a problem. Eventually Theresa was placed in a special education self-contained classroom. While she is not believed to be mentally retarded, the majority of her classmates were so classified. A short time later it was clear that she was having extreme difficulty in developing useful communication skills. She was failing to acquire language beyond primitive gestures. School officials concluded that the absence of other deaf children in the school program, the nature of the family constellation, and the lack of an alternative communication system for Theresa all contributed to a highly restrictive environment for her educational development. They believed the least restrictive environment was placement in the state-supported residential school for the deaf, where she could benefit from the association of other deaf children and learn sign language. A visit to the state school by the grandmother led her to support the plan.

Theresa is learning sign language at the state school and now communicates effectively with other deaf children, staff members, and her teachers at the school. Her academics are progressing nicely, although she is about 1 year behind her peers at the school. Teachers believe she will close the gap in time. Also important is the fact that the grandmother and other family members are trying to learn sign language so they can communicate with Theresa when she visits her home.

This case study shows that the least restrictive environment is a relative concept. Clearly the options for a meaningful, educational experience in this child's home district were unduly restrictive. While other educational alternatives exist, the IEP team with the support of the family prefers the state residential school.

Summary

Some Important Points to Remember

- Early detection and management of hearing loss can increase the potential for educational achievement and personal adjustment.
- The critical period for developing language occurs between 6 months and 4 years of age.
- A major goal for a child classified as hard of hearing is to learn spoken language.
- Methodologies for hard of hearing children stress properly fitting hearing aids, auditory training, language stimulation, and speech production training.
- Cued speech is not a sign language, but rather uses hand signals to provide cues about speech sounds that are produced but not lipreadable.
- The Rochester method uses fingerspelling of words that are being spoken.
- There is controversy about the appropriate use of auditory methods for children who have been classified as deaf.
- American Sign Language is a bona fide language in itself as it has its own vocabulary and grammar.
- Total communication is a philosophy that specifies that each deaf child be provided any combination of communication systems that facilitates learning and personal adjustment.
- Hearing aids are electronic devices that make sounds louder but do not provide hearing where residual hearing does not exist.
- Small hearing aids that are worn in the ear often present feedback problems when extra volume is needed for persons with significant losses because the microphone and receiver are too close to each other.
- School hearing screening tests do not show decibels of hearing loss.
- The only reliable method of identifying hearing loss is audiometric testing.
- Hard of hearing children are often mainstreamed, but many deaf children are not mainstreamed due to poor academic achievement.
- Children with hearing impairments essentially produce speech as they hear it.
- Hard of hearing children consistently show a 2-year lag in vocabulary development, and deaf children show about a 4- to 5-year lag.

"Do"s and "Don't"s for Teachers

"Do"s:

- Learn about the child's hearing aid.
- Be aggressive in achieving an ideal emotional climate for the child.
- Facilitate communication among all professionals working with the child.
- Be realistic in your academic expectations for the child; consult other school specialists for advice.
- Become familiar with the child's standardized test performance profile, especially language scores.
- Face the child during all oral communication.

- Frequently check with the child to make sure he or she is comprehending.
- Use appropriate visual teaching aids whenever practical.
- Become familiar with appropriate resource materials, and when practical order such materials for your classroom.
- Encourage the child to ask questions.
- Check with the speech-language pathologist or audiologist about the hearing-listening environment in the classroom.

"Don't"s:

- Do not hide the child's hearing problem; be honest and straightforward in dealing with the child's peers.
- Do not exaggerate pronunciation.

Referral Resources

- Audiologists
- Otologists
- Speech-language pathologists
- Hearing resource teachers
- Teachers for the learning disabled
- Clinical psychologists
- Neurologists

Self-Test

True or False:

1. Hard of hearing children are more frequently seen in classrooms than are deaf children.   _____

2. Hearing screening procedures utilize a pure tone audiometer to determine a child's ability to detect certain frequencies at preset levels.   _____

3. There are three definitive ways to recognize hearing loss in children simply by observing their behavior.   _____

4. As listening becomes more difficult, the hearing-impaired child will rely more on visual information.   _____

5. Good advice for the classroom teacher when communicating with hearing-impaired children is to exaggerate pronunciation.   _____

6. Children born with hearing loss show essentially the same types and magnitude of speech and language problems as those who acquire hearing loss after speech has developed.   _____

7. Children with hearing impairments often produce speech as they hear it.   _____

8. Data show that all deaf children demonstrate about a 2-year lag in vocabulary development.   _____

9. Almost all deaf children are mainstreamed into regular classrooms.   _____

10. Language disorders are rarely caused by hearing loss.   _____

11. Ability to localize sounds usually occurs around 3 to 5 months.   _____

12. All auditory methods require the study of lipreading.   _____

13. Cued speech is now considered the sign language of choice.   _____

14. Most professionals prefer oral methods over manual methods.   _____

15. Total communication includes the use of sign language.   _____

16. Many deaf adults prefer the use of sign language over auditory-oral communication.   _____

17. Various devices that help the deaf person understand the auditory events in the environment are called assistive listening devices.   _____

18. Auditory feedback is a common problem for children who wear hearing aids that fit entirely in the ear.   _____

19. The cochlear implant is the most recent type of hearing aid developed.   _____

20. Most persons with a hearing impairment can benefit from a cochlear implant.   _____

References

Alpiner, J., & McCarthy, P. (Eds.). (1993). *Rehabilitative audiology, children and Adults* (2nd ed.). Baltimore, MD: Williams & Wilkins.

Cornett, R. (1967). Cued speech. *American Annals of the Deaf, 121*, 3–13.

Crandell, C., & Smaldino, J. (1996). Sound-field amplification in the classroom: Applied and theoretical issues. In F. Bess, J. Gravel, & A. Tharpe (Eds.), *Amplification for children with auditory deficits* (pp. 229–250). Nashville, TN: Bill Wilkerson Center Press.

House, W. (1982). Surgical considerations in cochlear implants. *Annals of Otology, Rhinology, and Laryngology, 91*, 15–20.

Moores, D. (1987). *Educating the deaf: Psychology, principles, and practices.* Boston: Houghton Mifflin.

Ross, M., Brackett, D., & Maxon A. (1991). *Assessment and management of mainstreamed hearing-impaired children, principles and practices.* Austin, TX: Pro-Ed.

Schow, R., & Nerbonne, M. (Eds.). (1996). *Introduction to audiologic rehabilitation* (3rd ed.). Boston: Allyn & Bacon.

Tucker, J. D. (1997). *IDEA advocacy for children who are deaf or hard of hearing.* San Diego, CA: Singular Publishing Group.

C h a p t e r 8

Low-Incidence Populations and Techniques of Special Concern

Many children exhibit communication problems as part of a more involved disorder. With inclusion, you will eventually have these children in your classrooms. You may find them very challenging until you get to know them and their needs. One of the teacher's responsibilities is to have a basic understanding of some of the ramifications of these problems as they affect learning, communication, and social adjustment. Of great importance as well is for the teacher to have a close liaison with the parents of these children with special problems. Such a liaison can provide an insight into parent attitudes, the capabilities of the child as viewed by the parents, how the parents deal with problems of communication and learning at home, and the level of aspiration the parents hold for their child. The relationship also can have far-reaching effects for the child throughout adolescence and as the child/adolescent leaves the school setting.

Therefore, the purpose of this chapter is to expose you to some of these populations and to briefly describe some remediation techniques. Because the children will vary so much in the exact characteristics and severity of each of those characteristics, you will find that you will do "on-the-job training" with many of them. The disorders and techniques were chosen for discussion here based on teacher requests. We hope you will find working with these children a source of professional and personal satisfaction.

What Special Problems May the Teacher Encounter in the Classroom?

Head Injuries

Each year more than one million children and youth experience a traumatic brain injury (TBI) (Russell, 1993). TBIs are the leading cause of death in pediatric populations and are most apt to happen to males in their adolescent years (Chapman, 1997; Turkstra, 1999). A TBI may be either closed or open. A closed head injury is more common and involves a nonpenetrating wound to the brain, often as a result of an accident involving a car, truck, motorcycle, bicycle, and/or pedestrian; a fall, a sports injury, or child abuse. Open head injuries are the result of a penetrating wound to the brain, such as from a gunshot.

The outcome may be mild to severe depending on the severity of the injury and the location of the injury within the brain. Some of the problems caused by the brain injury will be temporary as brain swelling decreases and other parts of the brain have a chance to compensate for the part of the brain that was injured. Other problems will be permanent. Typical problems that you may encounter when the student returns to school include:

- Difficulty with short-term and/or long-term memory
- Slowness in thinking
- Confusion
- Distractibility, poor attention span
- Difficulty with word retrieval
- Poor judgment
- Difficulty processing information
- Difficulty with understanding an assignment, identifying the steps for completing the assignment, and carrying out the steps
- Personality changes including aggression, cussing, apathy, frustration, depression, mood swings, a short temper, and inappropriate sexual behaviors
- Physical difficulties with gross and/or fine motor movement, coordination, and strength
- Hearing loss
- Visual problems, ranging from blurred vision to a loss of part of the field of vision, double vision, and/or the loss of accommodation (the ability of the brain to combine the images from both eyes into one image with depth)
- Seizures
- Headaches
- Speech problems, such as slurred-sounding speech; the terms *dysarthria* or *apraxia* may be used
- Other receptive and expressive language difficulties, especially in the areas of syntax and pragmatics
- Perseveration (the repeating of words or activities that were once appropriate but due to a change in the situation are no longer appropriate, such as contin-

uing to give the same answer over and over when the class has moved on to other work)
- Swallowing difficulties
- Fatigue

It is easy to see how speech, language, hearing, and academics may all be affected. It has also been noted that with very young children some problems may not become evident until several years post-injury when the child is confronted with more complicated linguistic and academic tasks (Hux, Walker, & Sanger, 1996). Also, keep in mind that in determining the effects of a brain injury, the abilities before the injury must be factored in.

Simple instructions for helping the student until you get to know and understand that student's particular problems better include:

- Use simple rather than complex language.
- Use gestures or other visual cues to accompany what you say.
- Give instructions step by step.
- Help the student avoid stress and potentially frustrating situations.
- Allow time for the child to respond, in terms of both verbal responses and physically carrying out instructions.
- Encourage the use of any equipment that the child now needs.
- Participate in meetings with the parents and other professionals prior to the child's returning to school to obtain as much information as possible to assist in the child's transition back to school.

Fetal Alcohol Syndrome

Because you will come across the word *syndrome* many times in medical terminology, it should be defined. A syndrome is a group of characteristics that result from a common cause and cluster together to form a particular identifiable clinical picture.

Three in 1,000 babies have enough exposure to alcohol while in utero that they are born with fetal alcohol syndrome (FAS). Babies with less exposure to alcohol while in utero, but still enough to cause disabilities, although less marked than in FAS, are born with fetal alcohol effects (FAE). These children are characterized by low birth weight; small head size; craniofacial anomalies (abnormal skull and facial features), including small eyes and protruding or cupped ears; hypoplasia (incomplete or undeveloped tissue) of the mouth and nose; central nervous system dysfunction; and malformations of major organs. Because of these problems, they typically display several of the following: delayed motor development; mild to profound mental handicaps; language disabilities; learning disabilities; short attention span; hyperactivity; behavioral problems; auditory processing difficulties; hearing and visual problems; and, of course, academic problems. A case history of alcohol abuse helps to identify this child, when the school wonders what caused all of the child's problems. However, not all families are willing to admit to alcohol abuse. As with other children, strengths and needs are identified. Educational goals build on the strengths and address the needs.

Autistic Spectrum Disorders

Autism is called a spectrum disorder because of the wide range of characteristics that may be displayed in a variety of combinations as well as the fact that symptoms may be mild to severe. This variety has led to children being labeled as "autistic-like," having "high-functioning autism," or "low-functioning autism," or as having "autistic tendencies." Children with autism will have delays in several developmental areas along with distinguishing characteristics including:

- Intelligence: Approximately 60 percent of these children will have IQs below 50, although intelligence can be normal.
- Communication: Language development ranging from totally absent language to delayed; use of gestures to indicate needs; echolalia (the echoing or repeating of what was heard); ignoring of verbal stimuli.
- Behavior: Ranging from overly passive to overly active and aggressive; difficulty with changes in daily routines; may be ritualistic about personal routines, such as putting crayons back in a box in an exact order; short attention span; perseveration; self-stimulating behaviors, such as hand-flapping or rocking; lacking fear of real dangers so survival skills are diminished; inappropriate emotional behavior, such as crying or laughing; extreme distress often displayed by way of tantrums for no apparent reason; inappropriate attachment to objects.
- Play: Does not use toys in a typical manner; lacks imaginative play.
- Social Interaction: Spends time alone rather than with others; little interest in friends; difficulty with social graces (e.g., eye contact, smiling, laughing).
- Sensory Impairment: May be over- or undersensitive to stimuli.
- Motoric Abilities: Skilled motor functions will be affected; clumsiness.
- May possess an exceptional talent, perhaps for math or music; these are often featured in news stories.

Autism is life-long, has no cure, and is thought to be caused by neurological and biological differences in the brain, but so far no definitive cause of these differences is known. The fact that some families have more than one member with autism or a related disorder indicates that genetics may play a role. Indeed, genetic research has identified genes that may affect neurotransmitters in the brain, the immune system, or the developing nervous system of the embryo (McIntosh, 1998). Four times more males are affected ("Autism," 1994). There are no medical tests that can diagnose autism. Diagnosis is made through observations of behavior and generally takes place by 30 months of age, but this has not always been the case. In the past, autism has been confused with deafness as well as emotional, attentional, and communication disorders.

What kind of help is available? The kinds of help provided are based on the characteristics present. Needs should be identified and possible solutions explored; progress should be evaluated with changes in solutions made as necessary. Approaches to helping the student with autism should be coordinated across the home, school, and community. The teacher will be concerned about at least the following:

- A behavior modification plan
- Academic approaches (in general, highly structured programs with intensive use of visuals work well)
- Communication—may range from improving verbal abilities to use of alternative augmentative communication (discussed later in this chapter) with children who have difficulty learning functional speech
- Social skills
- Functional living skills, such as crossing a street safely, selecting and making purchases in a store, and asking for help when it is needed

Medications for problems like seizures, hyperactivity, anxiety, and so on may be prescribed. Other treatments, some of which are controversial, that have been tried include diet and vitamin therapy, auditory integration training, facilitated communication, and sensory integration.

Autism can be compared and contrasted to the following developmental disabilities. *Pervasive developmental disorders (PDD)* is a term used by the American Psychiatric Association to refer to a broad category of severe and pervasive impairments in several areas of development. The child with PDD does not meet the criteria for any of the more specific diagnoses. *Asperger's disorder* is characterized by disabilities in social interactions and restricted interests and activities. The IQ is in the average to above average range with no significant delay in language. *Rett's disorder* begins between 1 and 4 years of age, occurs only in girls, and is characterized by a period of normal development followed by a loss of abilities and repetitive hand movements that replace purposeful use of the hands.

Students with Tracheostomies and Ventilators

A tracheostomy is an opening through the neck into the trachea through which an indwelling tube is placed to assist breathing. A ventilator is one of several devices used to assist respiration and intensive positive pressure breathing. It may promote full expansion of the lungs, improve oxygenation, or control air pressure or volume. Such procedures and devices are required by students who have a variety of medical conditions, including severe craniofacial anomalies and high-level spinal cord injuries. These students will have difficulty speaking and may have difficulty swallowing.

Speech-wise, they will have difficulty controlling volume; they cannot always initiate speech when they want to; the time in which they can talk is short; the time in between speech efforts when they will be silent but still want to talk is long. Listeners must be patient and not usurp the student's turn to talk just because of the unintentional and uncontrollable silence. Listeners, especially younger ones, may also have trouble following what the person on a ventilator is trying to say because of the time it takes to express the thought. Teachers can help here by explaining to classmates that the child needs more time and by rephrasing what the child said so that the thought is coherently expressed and can be understood.

Dysphagia (swallowing problems) may be due to difficulty in coordinating swallowing with respiration. Coughing and gagging indicate trouble, and all teachers should be prepared. Find out what to do for your particular student from the parents, speech-language pathologist, or school nurse before confronted with the situation. The student may be on a modified diet (the consistency of food determines how easy it is to swallow) or may need to be in a particular position (e.g., head or chin held correctly) in order to swallow more easily.

Cerebral Palsy

Cerebral palsy is a motor function disorder that is permanent, nonprogressive, and due to brain damage prenatally (before birth), perinatally (near the time of birth), or shortly postnatally (after birth). The damage is often associated with premature or abnormal birth and a lack of oxygen to the brain. The neurological damage may be mild to severe and result in motor dysfunctions that are classified under the labels of *spasticity, athetosis, ataxia,* or *rigidity*. Respectively, each of these accounts for approximately 65 to 80 percent, 12 percent, 12 percent, and 7 percent of cerebral palsy cases (Gelfer, 1996). Spasticity, the most frequent form, is characterized by increased muscle tone with uncontrolled and involuntary muscle contractions. Athetosis is characterized by slow, writhing, involuntary, and continuous movements of the arms and legs. Rigidity involves stiffness and inflexibility due to involuntary, excessive, and continuous muscle contractions. Ataxia is characterized by a disturbance in the ability to coordinate movements and maintain balance. The site and extent of the brain damage determine which parts of the body are affected and to what degree. The physical aspects of some people with cerebral palsy are barely noticeable, while those of others are diffuse and severe.

Cerebral palsy can be accompanied by speech, language, hearing, and vision problems; seizures; varying IQs from above normal to severe mental handicap; and emotional problems. Again, depending on the extent and site of damage, the associated problems may not be present at all or one or all may be present. With regard to speech, some or all of the muscles associated with the processes necessary for speech production, that is, respiration, phonation (vocal fold action), resonance, and articulation, may be affected. Vowels as well as consonants may be affected. Facial grimaces, head movements, and other body movements that indicate neuromuscular incoordination and effort frequently accompany speech attempts.

The degree of involvement will dictate the needs of the child in the classroom. Speech-wise, the range extends from no involvement, to articulation problems, to the need for alternative augmentative communication. Language therapy, help from special education teachers, occupational therapy for fine motor movements, and physical therapy may or may not be necessary.

Down Syndrome

Down syndrome is the most common chromosomal abnormality, occurring in approximately 7 in every 1,000 births (Gerber, 1990). It is a congenital condition that is marked by a mental handicap, typically with IQ in the 50 to 60 range, and physical characteristics, including depressed nasal bridge; a slant to the eyes; low-set ears; a large, protruding tongue; short, broad hands with stubby fingers; and a shorter than average, stocky stature. Congenital heart disease, vision and hearing problems, and chronic respiratory infections are also often present. These children will need speech and language therapy. Some will need a form of alternative augmentative communication.

HIV and AIDS

Because of confidentiality, the child with HIV or AIDS may never be identified at school. However, 1 in 1,000 children is born with HIV, the virus that can be a precursor to acquired immune deficiency syndrome (AIDS) (Rabins, 1996). This child may also have been exposed to drugs in utero. Other children may acquire HIV or AIDS after birth, during their preschool or school-age years. Developmental delays, articulation disorders, language disabilities, dysphagia (swallowing difficulties), and hearing problems are common. In fact, chronic otitis media may well be one of the first symptoms, because the child's immune system will not let him or her fight off the organisms causing the ear infection (Boswell, 1999; Rabins, 1996). Also, some of the drugs used to treat HIV and AIDS are ototoxic, meaning that they cause hearing loss. Worse yet is the fact that as the disease progresses, abilities may decline.

Central Auditory Processing Difficulties

Children with central auditory processing difficulties do not have a peripheral hearing loss and an audiogram will appear normal. However, they act as if they have a hearing loss. They often do not respond to questions, do not follow instructions, and are inattentive. The problem may be mild to severe. Academic failure may lead to a learning disability or attention deficit disorder label. The problem lies within the auditory cortex of the brain; these children hear but have difficulty (1) processing or attaching meaning to what they hear and (2) remembering what they hear, especially if the message is long, complex, spoken rapidly or if background noises or visual distractions are present. However, one on one in a distraction-free environment, these children do quite well. Speech-language therapy may involve auditory training, mnemonics to improve the memory, and exercises to improve the ability to pay attention. In the classroom an assistive listening device to improve the signal-to-noise ratio (think of this as the relative loudness of the noise to be heeded, in this case the teacher's voice, to other irrelevant noise), preferential seating near the teacher, and compensatory techniques can make a significant difference.

What Remediation Techniques Are Available for Children with Special Problems?

Alternative Augmentative Communication

An alternative or augmentative communication device is anything that enables a person who cannot communicate in the "normal" manner to communicate in other ways (Radcliffe, Cress, & Soto, 1997). Alternative devices are just that—an alternative, whereas augmentative devices involve a medium that supplements rather than replaces natural speech (Gelfer, 1996). All sorts of individuals are candidates for alternative augmentative communication. Those with hearing impairments, autism, physical handicaps such as cerebral palsy and paralysis (loss of muscle function), mental handicaps, Down syndrome, or brain damage from injuries or strokes are just a few examples (Glennen & DeCoste, 1996).

The communication device may be as simple as a communication board consisting of a piece of cardboard with pictures of family members and other children in the classroom, the letters of the alphabet, toys, food, bathroom, or anything else that a child might want or need to communicate about. There may be more than one communication board for use in different settings, such as home, the cafeteria, the classroom during reading, the classroom during mathematics, and the playground. On the playground the communication board might be cut into smaller pieces, hole punched, and put together with a metal loop that can hang from the child's clothing for easy access while leaving the hands free for play. A slightly more sophisticated device would be a low-tech device that has speech output based on preprogrammed messages, such as "Would you like to play?" or "I'm tired." A considerably more sophisticated and costly device would be a computer with various adaptations for the child who has a physical disability as well as a communication disability. The adaptations might include a headstick that is attached to the head and operated by moving the head, light-controlled switches, or pneumatic switches. Software might include a word prompt or prediction capability program that guesses at the correct word when the student types in just the first few letters, speech/voice recognition programs, or speech synthesis.

Dedicated systems are technological devices intended for use by persons with communication and physical disabilities. With increased portability, more and more individuals are selecting "regular" computers and adding adaptations, such as alternative keyboards, switching devices for use with Morse code, and touch window capabilities. These computers can also more readily provide electronic access to programs, such as encyclopedias and other reference materials.

Choosing the appropriate system and the vocabulary needed involves determining what the student needs to be able to communicate and how this might best be accomplished. Letters, words, symbols, pictures, photographs, and line drawings are all options for use as communication symbols. Physical and mental capabilities must be considered, because the child needs to be able physically to use the device and to be able mentally to understand how to use it. Funding is a problem for the higher-tech devices. The speech-language pathologist may spend quite a bit of time shadowing and working with children to determine their needs. All teachers should have lots of input and ideas about what the child needs to communicate and what would improve quality of life. For example, the music teacher might want to be able to program in the verses of songs so that the child can "sing" along. The teacher who directs high school plays might ask for a program that can produce sound effects so that the student can participate in drama productions. A teacher might want to be able to program in vocabulary that will be used in upcoming lessons.

Once a device is selected, the child and all of the communication partners (teachers, parents, classmates) need to learn how to use the device. The speech-language pathologist will provide the training, regularly assess how well it is working, and provide any needed services. The goal is for the student to be able to express the same sorts of thoughts that other students do and to be able to participate in the same activities (e.g., academics, extracurricular activities, small talk, and making friends). How this is done will change as the child grows older. To begin with, communication boards and low-tech devices are very appropriate, but later, as the child grows and develops cognitively and more is expected academically, more sophisticated capabilities are needed and, thus, high-tech equipment is frequently the best option.

Signing (considered a total language) is another form of alternative augmentative communication. There are several kinds of sign language. American Sign Language (ASL) is used by the deaf community. Signing Exact English (SEE), which allows for morphemes to be added, is also frequently used in the schools, especially by children who are not hearing impaired or who have as a goal learning to speak as the primary means of expressive communication. The major drawbacks of signing are that (1) it limits communication partners to those who know some sign and (2) younger children and those with fine motor problems may have difficulty moving the fingers to form some of the signs.

Signing is sometimes used with children, in particular children with Down syndrome, as a means of teaching language and communication until the child learns to speak. Thus, a child may come to school using a combination of verbal communication and sign. Other children, such as those with hearing impairments, will be taught sign as a life-long form of communication. The classroom teacher may be expected to learn some signs. However, if this is the primary mode of communication, a sign language interpreter will be necessary. The speech-language pathologist or interpreter may teach signs in the child's classroom so that the child's classmates and the child will have a way to communicate with each other. Interestingly, some research has shown that the use of isolated signs can help all children learn to read better (Peters-Johnson, 1995b). The sign adds another visual input for words that are hard to remember. When any of your students is having difficulty learning to read a word (perhaps a sight word that cannot be sounded out), ask the speech-language pathologist for the sign for that word and try using it. Many signs resemble the words that they stand for. If you are still in college or will attend, note that some colleges and universities allow students to meet a for eign language requirement by taking sign language classes.

Cued Speech

Cued speech is an alternative means of visual communication that was devised to help prelingually deaf (deaf prior to learning language) children improve language and reading abilities. It has been described as a visual phonetic analog of speech. Hand cues and lip movements are used to distinguish vowels and consonants. It has also been used with children who have PDD, autism, auditory processing difficulties, reading disabilities, and mental handicaps. (See also the discussion of cued speech with hard of hearing children in Chapter 7.)

Sensory Integration Therapy

Many children with disabilities like cerebral palsy, mental handicaps, attention deficit disorder, autism spectrum disorders, Down syndrome, and central nervous system disorders have difficulty organizing sensory information so that they can understand what is happening to them and learn about the world around them. Of concern is visual, auditory, tactile, kinesthetic, vestibular, and proprioceptive input. These children may exhibit gravitational insecurity, visual discrimination problems, or tactile or auditory hypersensitivities. A child with a tactile hypersensitivity is also described as "tactile defensive" and will not be comfortable with touching or being touched. A child with auditory hypersensitivities will be disturbed by noises that are ignored by classmates. The occupational therapist is the professional who plans sensory integration therapy and will provide other educational personnel with the information they need to understand and carry out therapy plans.

Auditory Integration Training

Auditory integration training (AIT) is highly controversial. Many look upon it askance. Because of anecdotal reports of improvements, many call for more research in this area. There are three recognized auditory integration training methods: Tomatis, Clark, and Berard (Peters-Johnson, 1995a). The training is based on the assumption that the auditory system is directly related to attention and behavior and that changes in attention and behavior will occur if the auditory system can be reorganized through listening treatments (Madell & McPherson, 1997). Treatments consist of listening to a music or speech signal that has passed through an auditory training device. These devices, which are regulated by the Federal Drug Administration as medical devices, manipulate the frequency and/or intensity of the signal.

This procedure has been used in other countries, primarily France and Canada, with learning disabilities, but in the United States it has been used with many disorders, including autism, depression, dyslexia, suicidal tendencies, hearing loss, tinnitus (ringing in one or both ears), pervasive developmental delay, learning problems, epilepsy, and even premenstrual syndrome (Madell & McPherson, 1997; Rimland & Edelson, 1994).

Frequency-Modulated Systems

The use of frequency-modulated (FM) systems and auditory trainers has been standard for students with hearing losses for many years. There are several devices available, primarily divided into personal FM systems and sound field amplification systems. They all work by improving the signal-to-noise ratio in environments that are noisy and reverberant. In this context, noise can be defined as any sound that interferes with the signal that should be heard (Position Statement and Guidelines for Acoustics in Educational Settings, 1995). At school, noise may originate in the classroom or from outside of the classroom. Reverberation is the process of sounds being reflected repeatedly and interfering with the signal that should be heard. The amount of reverberation increases with room size and decreases when there are sound-absorbing materials present, such as carpeting and other softer materials. Typically classrooms are noisy environments and are more apt to have surfaces, such as concrete walls, that increase reverberation.

Even children with normal hearing may benefit from amplification systems (Johnson et al., 1997). However, children with language disabilities, learning disabilities, attention deficit disorders, and auditory processing difficulties can especially benefit from a clearer signal. Teacher fatigue may also be reduced when children attend better.

Facilitated Communication

Facilitated communication is a technique in which another person called a facilitator assists a person with a severe communication disability to communicate through pointing, eye gaze, or other means. The facilitator determines, often from very little information from the person with the disability, what it is that the person would communicate if able. This has been a very controversial means of communication because, to date, research has shown that the communication does not appear to originate with the person with the disability but rather with the facilitator. There is also concern that with facilitated communication being used, no other more appropriate communication method may be tried.

General Comments

There are so many problems that can cause potential speech, language, and hearing problems that will in turn affect academic success that it is not feasible to discuss them all within one book. For example, there are children exposed to drugs in utero, children with lead poisoning, children with various other syndromes not discussed in this book, and children who are emotionally and/or physically abused. It should be pointed out that children with severe disabilities are at high risk for abuse. Often they are unable to tell anyone about the abuse; however, unexplained changes in behavior may signal the need to ask questions. Also, symptoms of abuse are often attributed to the disability.

This introduction to some of the low-incidence populations should give you a basis for being able to generalize your knowledge to other infrequently encountered conditions. Whatever problems that the children in your classrooms present, remember that you are in a position to do a world of good or cause unnecessary hurt. The medical profession, the home, and the school need to work together as a team. The school is responsible for medical management during the school day, for identifying the academic strengths and weaknesses of the child, and for working on those weaknesses within the context of the regular curriculum and the regular classroom if at all possible. Most of all, remember that these children are children who need to be loved and respected no matter what problems they have. They also need to learn to laugh and enjoy life. How to enjoy and occupy leisure time is a goal that many more IEP committees need to consider, especially for children who present multiple or severe disabilities.

Summary

Some Important Points to Remember

- Head injuries are most apt to happen to males during their adolescent years.
- TBIs may be either closed or open.
- Perseveration means the repeating of a word(s) or activity(ies) that was once appropriate but is no longer appropriate because the situation has changed.
- Finding out from the parents and professionals who have worked with a child who has had a TBI what problems to expect and how to handle them prior to the child returning to school is helpful to both the child and the school staff.
- The word *syndrome* refers to a group of characteristics that result from a common cause and cluster together to form a particular identifiable clinical picture.
- Most children with autism have a mental handicap.
- Children with autism typically do not handle changes in routine easily.
- Self-stimulating behaviors and a lack of social interaction are common in children with autism.
- Autism, pervasive developmental delay, Rett's disorder, and Asperger's syndrome belong to the same spectrum of disorders.
- An alternative communication device provides an alternative to normal verbal communication.
- Augmentative communication is a supplement to verbal communication.
- Alternative augmentative communication may involve pictures, letters, printed words, symbols, photographs, and line drawings used with no-tech, low-tech, or high-tech devices as well as sign language.
- A preprogrammed computer with voice output may be used to help a child fit in with peers in both academic and extracurricular activities.
- Students with tracheostomies and ventilators will have a great deal of difficulty talking and may have swallowing problems as well.

- Cerebral palsy is due to brain damage involving the motor areas of the brain and may involve other areas of the brain as well, causing sensory and/or intellectual deficits.
- In cerebral palsy, if the damaged motor areas of the brain involve the muscles that support speech, the ability to speak will be impaired.
- Children with Down syndrome typically have a mental handicap and a recognizable set of physical characteristics.
- Chronic otitis media may be one of the first symptoms of HIV.
- Children with central auditory processing difficulties can have normal peripheral hearing and thus a normal audiogram, but have difficulty in the brain with processing auditory input.
- Children with a variety of disabilities may have difficulty using sensory information to learn about the world.
- Auditory integration training is a controversial procedure.
- Research does not support facilitated communication.
- FM systems may provide ideal hearing environments for many students.
- When writing IEPs, especially for children with many problems and who may never be able to hold a job, be sure to think about how children can best communicate and learn to enjoy life, including having fun and occupying leisure time.

Self-Test

True or False:

1. Approximately 500,000 children and youth experience a traumatic brain injury each year.   _____

2. The problems that some very young children have after traumatic brain injuries may not show up until years later when they are expected to deal with more complicated linguistic and academic tasks.   _____

3. *Dysarthria* refers to slurred-sounding speech.   _____

4. Over one-half of the children with autism will have a mental handicap.   _____

5. A child with autism may be a candidate for alternative augmentative communication.   _____

6. Signing is used as a substitute for talking, not as a means of teaching language.   _____

7. A syndrome is a group of characteristics, each of which may be due to a variety of causes.   _____

8. Hearing and visual problems are characteristics of fetal alcohol syndrome.   _____

9. A ventilator is an opening through the neck into the trachea through which an indwelling tube is placed to assist breathing.   _____

10. Ventilator-assisted speech is often slow and characterized by uncontrolled volume. _____

11. *Dysesophagus* refers to swallowing problems. _____

12. Cerebral palsy generally starts after age 2. _____

13. Spasitosis is one form of cerebral palsy in which there is increased muscle tone. _____

14. Not all children with cerebral palsy will have articulation problems. _____

15. The most common chromosomal disorder is Down syndrome. _____

16. Alternative augmentative communication is useful with some children who have Down syndrome. _____

17. Some HIV drugs are ototoxic. _____

18. Signal-to-noise ratio refers to the teacher alerting a child with a hearing loss that instructions are about to be given and that the child should listen carefully. _____

19. Cued speech was developed with prelingually deaf children but has also been used with children who have PDD, autism, reading disabilities, and auditory processing difficulties. _____

20. Children who are tactile defensive like to touch everything within reach. _____

21. Research has shown that auditory integration training works well with most children who are hearing impaired. _____

22. Reverberation is a technique for working with children who have tinnitus. _____

23. The child with central auditory processing difficulties will do better when working one on one than when there is a noisy background. _____

24. Facilitated communication is the ideal solution for children who have both physical and communication handicaps. _____

25. No matter what the child's problem is, the IEP committee must identify the child's strengths and needs and use the strengths to address the child's needs while teaching the regular educational curriculum within the regular classroom, if at all possible. _____

References

Autism. (1994). *ASHA, 36,* 83.

Boswell, S. (1999). Probing HIV/AIDS link to communication disorders. *ASHA Leader, 4*(1), 1, 6.

Chapman, S. B. (1997). Cognitive-communication abilities in children with closed head injury. *American Journal of Speech-Language Pathology, 6,* 50–58.

Gelfer, M. (1996). *Survey of communication disorders.* New York: McGraw-Hill.

Gerber, S. E. (1990). Chromosomes and chromosomal disorders. *ASHA, 32*(9), 39.

Glennen, S., & DeCoste, D. (1996). *The handbook of augmentative and alternative communication.* San Diego, CA: Singular Publishing Group.

Hux, K., Walker, M., & Sanger, D. D. (1996). Traumatic brain injury: Knowledge and self-perceptions of school speech-language pathologists. *Language, Speech, and Hearing Services in Schools, 27,* 171–184.

Johnson, C. E., Stein, R. L., Broadway, A., & Markwalter, T. S. (1997). "Minimal" high-frequency hearing loss and school-age children: Speech. *Language, Speech, and Hearing Services in Schools, 28,* 77–85.

Madell, J. R., & McPherson, D. L. (1997). Auditory integration training: What's next? *ASHA, 39*(1), 10–11.

McIntosh, H. (1998). Autism is likely to be linked to several genes. *The Monitor, 29,* 13.

Peters-Johnson, C. (1995a). Auditory integration training. *Language, Speech, and Hearing Services in Schools, 26,* 108–109.

Peters-Johnson, C. (1995b). Signing helps all kids.

Language, Speech, and Hearing Services in Schools, 26, 301.

Position Statement and Guidelines for Acoustics in Educational Settings (1995). *ASHA,* March 1995, Suppl. 14, pp. 15.

Rabins, A. (1996). Convention '95. *ASHA Leader, 1*(1), 1, 3.

Radcliffe, A., Cress, C., & Soto, G. (1997). Communication isn't just talking. *ASHA, 39*(2), 30–36.

Rimland, B., & Edelson, S. M. (1994). The effects of auditory integration training on autism. *American Journal of Speech-Language Pathology, 3,* 16–24.

Russell, N. K. (1993). Educational considerations in traumatic brain injury: The role of the speech-language pathologist. *Language, Speech, and Hearing Services in Schools, 24,* 67–75.

Turkstra, L. S. (1999). Language testing in adolescents with brain injury: A consideration of the CELF-3. *Language, Speech, and Hearing Services in Schools, 30,* 132–140.

Chapter 9

Teachers and Their Responsibilities Regarding Communication

It has been emphasized throughout this book that the classroom teacher has a tremendous impact on children in general and especially on children with communicative problems. There is no doubt that teachers have busy schedules and little time for extra duties; however, teachers do have a number of responsibilities in relation to communication. First, there are the duties that are specified in the IEPs of the children who have communication disabilities in their classrooms. Second, there are some general responsibilities concerning communication. Teachers should find that, as they become more involved in and knowledgeable about communication, less time will be required for these responsibilities, and it is hoped that, as children learn to communicate better, the teachers will feel that the time spent was worthwhile.

General Responsibilities of a Teacher

The following general responsibilities will hold true regardless of the communicative situation or disorder.

Be a Good Speech Model

By being a good speech model the teacher subtly tells students that good communication is desirable. If you have any doubts whatsoever about your own communicative status, seek out a speech-language pathologist who can evaluate your speech. If you are a student, determine if there is a speech and hearing science department at your college or university. This specialty may be a separate department or it may be a part of a larger department, such as communications or special education. If you locate one, call and ask how you can obtain an evaluation. If you do have a problem, there probably is a clinic at which you can receive help at no cost or for a nominal fee. If you are reading this book as part of a course, you might also ask your instructor if he or she is qualified to assess your speech skills. If you are already a teacher, you may wish to talk to the speech-language pathologist who serves your school. He or she can assess your speech as well as give you suggestions for remediating any problems.

Moreover, a teacher or prospective teacher does not want to maintain a correctable behavior that would be a potential source of teasing or name calling by students. Realistically, children may be wonderful to work with, but children do not just tease other children; at times they also tease or find names to call teachers behind their backs. Do not provide them with an easy target. Furthermore, parents may object to obvious communicative problems.

Create a Classroom Atmosphere Conducive to Communication

A relaxed atmosphere in which children are expected to be attentive listeners and respect what others say is conducive to communication. The verbally shy child should be provided an opportunity and encouraged to participate orally. The goal is for children to view communication as fun.

Note that if you want a classroom in which everyone listens to the person talking, just expecting children to be attentive listeners may not be enough. Active listening may need to be taught. Truesdale (1990) developed whole-body listening lessons in which children are taught to be active rather than passive listeners. Whole-body listening involves using your brain to think about what is heard, using your eyes to look at the speaker, keeping your mouth quiet (no talking, no eating or chewing gum), keeping your hands still, keeping your feet still, and sitting tall with your seat on your chair or your spot on the floor.

Accept a Child with Communicative Problems

Truly accept a child as he or she is, remembering that there is a difference between acceptance and tolerance. Understand that a child may not be able to produce the "correct" speech behavior just because he or she is told or ordered to do so; the child may not even hear the difference between his or her speech and the "correct" speech. Be assured that the speech-language pathologist will inform the teacher when a child can be expected to use new communicative behaviors outside of therapy.

Encourage Classmates to Accept a Child with Communicative Problems

There is little doubt that a child's ability to communicate may affect how he or she is treated by peers, which may in turn affect the child's communication and willingness to communicate. No teacher can ever prevent or stop all teasing, or make children befriend other children; however, there are some strategies that may be helpful.

The school counselor may be able to provide you with materials or come into the classroom for some lessons involving feelings, attitudes, and lifeskills, such as caring. Make use of such opportunities whenever possible, not only for the benefit of the child with a communication disability but also for children who are doing the teasing, because they need to learn more acceptable adult behaviors. Appendix A includes an annotated bibliography of children's books, with either calculated readability levels or suggested grade levels, that deal with communicative problems as well as normal communication. The teacher may find some of these books appropriate for either individual readers or for the whole class.

When classmates have questions about a child with a disability, it may be appropriate to discuss the child's problems and how the other children can help. Depending on the circumstances, it may be more appropriate to hold this discussion with or without the child with the disability being present. However, the teacher might be wise to first discuss this approach and the reasons for it with the child's parents so that the parents will not learn of such a discussion through the "parental grapevine." We were particularly impressed with the mother of a severely physically disabled but completely mainstreamed child who came to class and, with her child, discussed what the child's problems were, how she coped with everyday activities, and how the classroom children could help. They then answered all questions.

At other times a teacher may need to help a child "fight back." For example, a third-grade girl was being mercilessly teased by a pair of sixth-grade boys in the hallways and on the playground. After considering the situation in terms of what would be most repugnant to boys of that age, the teacher remarked to the girl that when a boy teases a girl, it often means that he likes her. That afternoon as the boys confronted the girl, the girl yelled, "Boys who like girls tease them," and kept shouting it as she chased them across the playground. From then on, the boys avoided that little girl! Not all of your attempts may turn out as well, but you can at least try. Mercer and Mercer (1985) suggest that a teacher counsel children who are teased to ignore their tormentors, and then reward the teased children when they do ignore the teasing. In this way the child doing the teasing receives no attention from either the children being teased or the teacher.

Consult and Collaborate with the Speech-Language Pathologist

All school personnel have a responsibility to understand the goals and procedures being used by others who are working with a particular child and to work to integrate those goals and procedures into their own work with the child. This can only be accomplished by taking the time to explain what you are doing; listening to others explain what they are doing; and working out compatible goals, objectives, materials, and procedures. This is a major goal of the IEP committee. However, even after the IEP has been established, the consultation and collaboration must continue for daily and weekly problems to be worked out and goals to be accomplished. For example, with the traditional pullout service delivery model the classroom teacher can ask the speech-language pathologist to help the child with a particular task that the child is having difficulty with in the classroom, and the speech-language pathologist can ask the teacher to remind a child to use a particular language structure that the child has worked on in therapy. Obviously, with the classroom-based service delivery model, consultation and collaboration would be constant.

Furthermore, a teacher's knowledge and understanding of other services that a child receives, such as speech therapy, are also helpful when parents, who typically have more communication with the classroom teacher than with the speech-language pathologist, ask the teacher questions about such services. The teacher may be able to answer the questions but, if not, can at least talk knowledgeably about the questions while suggesting that the parents contact the speech-language pathologist, or, better yet, offering to have the speech-language pathologist contact the parents. A teacher should share information that may affect a child's performance or interaction with others. For example, because of more contact with the parents, a teacher may be better able to assess the parents' interest, willingness, or ability to help a child with his or her speech at home.

Detect Possible Communicative Problems and Make Appropriate Referrals to a Speech-Language Pathologist

When teachers detect possible speech or language problems, they should make referrals to a speech-language pathologist. Most speech-language pathologists will agree that they would prefer that teachers overrefer rather than underrefer so that children, especially those with subtle language problems and voice problems, are not missed. Generally school districts will have referral forms available in the principal's office. On these forms (see Figure 9-1) a teacher may be asked to describe the

XYZ SCHOOL DISTRICT
SPEECH-LANGUAGE-HEARING REFERRAL FORM

Student Name _____   Date _____

Age _____   Grade _____

Gender _____   School Building _____

Current Placement and Services _____

Referring Teacher _____

Check the area(s) that you are concerned about:

❑ Articulation/Production of Speech Sounds   ❑ Voice

❑ Stuttering/Fluency   ❑ Language

❑ Hearing   ❑ Other

Please describe the student's communicative problem. (Include frequency of problem and times/situations when problem is most noticeable.)

Please describe any technique(s) that have been tried in the classroom to address this problem and the success achieved:

Any other pertinent information:

FIGURE 9-1   Sample form for referral to speech-language pathologist.

problem and to state how he or she has attempted to deal with it and with what success. However, this does not preclude a teacher talking directly with the speech-language pathologist about a child.

Contribute to the Child's Motivation

Motivating a child is always important. Therapy is not something done to a child but instead requires cooperative effort on the child's part. Children need support from parents, teachers, and important others in their environment in order to put forth the effort to be a part of the remediation team. When two or more problems coexist creating a more complex disorder, motivation is particularly important, as therapy is not only apt to be long-term, but progress may be slow and "normal" may never be achievable.

Long before teachers can reinforce new communicative behaviors, they can encourage and motivate children through their interest in what the children are doing in therapy. Ask each child what he or she is learning. If the child has a "speech book," ask to see it and have the child tell you about it.

Reinforce the Goals of Speech Therapy

When a speech-language pathologist and teacher have consulted with each other, the teacher is in a position to reinforce the goals and procedures of speech therapy. As children progress and become capable of producing correct speech or language behaviors (whether it is a good "r" sound, a better voice quality, or a complete sentence), they must break old habit patterns and habituate new behaviors. This is the carryover stage during which a teacher can truly reinforce the new behavior. The speech-language pathology recognizes that the teacher is not trained in speech-language pathology and does not expect the teacher to hear or correct every error. In fact, having every error corrected could quickly discourage and alienate a child. However, there will be times when a teacher is aware that a child is using better speech or language. When this happens, the teacher should praise the child by saying, "You remembered to use your good 's' sound," or "Your voice certainly sounds better this morning." Remember, though, that such remarks in front of other children might embarrass a child. If you think this might be so, praise the child in private.

Help the Child Remember Therapy Appointments

This may be as simple as pointing out to a child that every Monday, Tuesday, and Thursday after recess, he or she should go to speech therapy. However, a visual reminder may be necessary. For example, a small clock with the hands pointing to the therapy time could be taped to a child's desk, or inside the desk if it needs to be inconspicuous. It is suggested that this be a clock face rather than the written time so that a child can match the reminder to the clock on the classroom wall.

Some children, whether due to impaired cognitive functioning or to other reasons, will not remember their therapy times regardless of what visual clues a teacher or speech-language pathologist provides. If such children are to get to therapy on time, the teacher must assume responsibility for remembering and reminding. Such help will be a tremendous benefit to the speech-language pathologist and to the children. If a child does not arrive at therapy on time, the speech-language pathologist will need to go personally or to send another child to the classroom to get the tardy child. This shortens the therapy time for all of the children. Similarly, a teacher certainly has the right to expect that children will be dismissed and sent back to the classroom on time.

Help the Child Catch Up on What Is Missed While in Speech Therapy

Whenever possible, a speech-language pathologist will schedule each child for the same time each day that the child attends therapy sessions in order to make it easier for the child (and the teacher) to remember that time. Therefore, it is suggested that teachers consider implementing (if they have not already done so) the currently popular practice of scheduling various subjects at different times each day. In this way a child will not be missing the same subject matter every therapy day.

Scheduling becomes more complicated at the secondary level because class schedules are more inflexible and the length of therapy sessions may not equal the length of class periods. Frequently attempts are made to schedule students during study halls, but this is impossible for all students. Rotating schedules may be used, but this approach makes it a bit more difficult for a student to remember therapy times. Scheduling speech therapy as part of the regular academic schedule for which students may earn credit has been suggested and tried in some school districts with success.

A teacher may want to spend some extra time with a child, reviewing subject matter missed during therapy. An alternative or additional technique would be to use a form of peer tutoring. The teacher would select a peer who would be responsible for explaining and reviewing the lessons and activities that the child missed. This peer might rotate according to the subject matter missed and might also rotate throughout the semester or year. If note taking is involved, the peer could photocopy or lend his or her notes. This might even be a part of a larger peer tutoring system within the classroom. It is beyond the scope of this book to delve into peer tutoring. However, studies have demonstrated it to be useful with benefits to both the tutors and tutees.

Prevention of Communication Disabilities

For communication disabilities, prevention should include providing information about general health issues and prenatal care so that children may be born with as few risk factors as possible. For example, not all people realize that alcohol, drugs, tobacco, lack of nutrients, and poor prenatal medical care can put newborns at risk for developmental disabilities. Once children are born, their exposure to communication practices may affect communicative status. Adults need to talk to children, read to children, and stimulate their speech and language development through techniques such as:

- Modeling: Restating what the child said in a slightly more advanced or mature manner. This might involve correcting a verb tense or an irregular plural, stressing a misarticulated sound in one of the words, etc.
- Expansion: Adding information to a child's utterance so that the language or vocabulary is slightly more advanced. For example, an adjective or adverb or a "because" clause might be added to the child's original utterance.
- Self-Talk: Talking about what you are doing as you are doing it. This can not only provide the child with the vocabulary to describe what you are doing, but you can also give the reason for doing what you are doing.
- Parallel Talk: Talking about what the child is doing while he or she is doing it.
- Cloze Technique: Starting the utterance and letting the child fill in the rest. For example, "Another name for a car is _____."

Children also need to be kept safe from a multitude of potentially harmful factors, including lead poisoning, accidents (through use of proper car seats, seat belts, helmets, etc.), physical and emotional abuse, voice abuse and misuse, and exposure to loud noises (including toys) without proper hearing protection.

Teachers have many opportunities to incorporate some of these issues into the curriculum either in whole-class lessons or as an individual paper or project. Think about a parenting class, a health class, a science class, a psychology class, a vocal hygiene program, or a hearing conservation program. What is it you could teach? There are many available resources, starting with your school's speech-language pathologist, who might teach a unit for you. Also, a good resource is the American Speech-Language-Hearing Association at 10801 Rockville Pike, Rockville, MD 20852 or call toll-free at (800) 638-8255 or (888) 321-ASHA. There are organizations for almost every disability relating to communication and education. Many organizations also have a certain time of year in which they publicize how they can help. For example, May is Better Speech and Hearing Month.

Summary

Some Important Points to Remember

- The classroom teacher is an important role model for children and thus is important in shaping their development.
- A teacher should become involved in a child's program of speech therapy.
- Being a good speech-language model tells children that good communication is highly desirable.
- If you, as a future teacher, think you have a speech problem, have your speech checked by a speech-language pathologist.

- An atmosphere conducive to easy communication should be established and maintained in the classroom.
- Show genuine acceptance of the child with a communicative disorder.
- The speech-language pathologist will inform a teacher when a child can be expected to use new communicative behaviors outside of therapy sessions; wait for this notification before demanding corrected speech-language behavior.
- Encourage classmates to accept a child with communicative disorders.
- Consult with the speech-language pathologist concerning each child with a communicative disorder in your classroom.
- Reinforce the goals of speech therapy.
- Reinforce good speech-language performance.
- Help children remember the times that they go to speech therapy.
- Be conscientious about helping children catch up on the classroom information they missed while in therapy.
- Consider peer tutoring to get children caught up on the classroom information they missed while in speech therapy sessions.
- Incorporate at least once a semester material(s) into your teaching plans that will help prevent communicative problems.

Questions to Ask Yourself

1. Name at least four ways that a classroom teacher can be a good speech model.
2. Develop a list that contains ten suggestions for developing an accepting atmosphere in the classroom for children with speech, language, or hearing impairments.
3. What role do parents play in the remediation process for their communicatively disabled child? At home? At school?
4. How might you, as a teacher, reinforce the work of a speech-language pathologist with a speech-disabled child in your classroom?
5. How might the speech-language pathologist reinforce the work you are doing in the classroom with a language-disabled child?
6. Elaborate on the concept of peer tutoring in either the elementary or secondary classroom for the child who must miss classroom activities to participate in speech therapy sessions.
7. Develop a lesson plan about prevention. Start by requesting literature from a national agency that advocates for a particular problem.

References

Mercer, C. D., & Mercer, A. R. (1985). *Teaching students with learning problems* (2nd ed.). Columbus, OH: Merrill.

Truesdale, S. P. (1990). Whole-body listening: Developing active auditory skills. *Language, Speech, and Hearing Disorders in Schools, 21,* 183–184.

Appendix *A*

Children's Literature Books Useful to Teachers

The books in this section are all suitable for your students. The readability level of each book (when appropriate) is listed just before the description. The readability levels were determined by a formula worked out by Fry (E. Fry, 1968, "A Readability Formula That Saves Time," *Journal of Reading, 11*, 513–516, 575–578). The books are arranged alphabetically by the last name of the first author.

These books were written for children and deal with the normal processes of speech and hearing and/or with impaired speech and hearing. It is hoped that teachers will be able to use them in some of the following ways: as part of a literature-based reading program, as supplements to science and health curricula, as recommended books for students doing book reports, as books to be read by the teacher to the entire class, as a supplement to discussions concerning feelings, and as suggested reading for individual students to either help them understand others' disabilities or to put their own disabilities into a better and healthier perspective. May your reading be enjoyable and informative!

Adams, B. (1979), *Like it is: Facts and feelings about handicaps from kids who know*. New York: Walker and Co. (96 pages) (approximate **7th grade readability** level)

This book portrays real children who reflect a variety of disabilities. They share with the reader factual information as well as their feelings about their disabilities. The purpose is to help readers become more comfortable and natural in their contacts with disabled peers. Thirteen-year-old Danny, who is deaf, talks about hearing and speech problems. Other chapters include children with visual impairments, orthopedic handicaps, developmental disabilities, learning disabilities, and behavior disorders. A glossary is included.

Adler, D. A. (1980). *Finger spelling fun*. New York: Franklin Watts. (32 pages) (approximate **4th grade readability** level)

Fingerspelling is defined and explained. The finger positions are depicted for each letter and the author suggests that they can be used as a secret code as well as for talking to deaf people. Riddles with answers given in fingerspelling will attract the young reader. Also included are games that utilize fingerspelling.

Adler, I., & Adler, R. (1963). *Your ears*. New York: John Day. (48 pages) (approximate **4th grade readability** level)

Beginning with a definition of sound, this book explains how we hear; how having two ears helps us localize sound; and how the ear is protected from dirt, unequal air pressure on either side of the eardrum, and very loud noises. Hearing tests, types of hearing loss, and various forms of remediation for the hearing impaired are also discussed.

Aimar, C. (1975). *Waymond the whale*. Englewood Cliffs, NJ: Prentice-Hall. (28 pages) (approximate **2nd grade readability** level)

Raymond and Elizabeth are brother and sister whales. Because of their speech problems they call each other Lithabeth and Waymond. They challenge each other to a contest but wind up helping each other learn to pronounce their sounds correctly.

Arthur, C., & Tablot, N. (1979). *My sister's silent world*. Chicago: Children's Press. (31 pages) (approximate **2nd grade readability** level)

This is a book of short narrative descriptions of a child, Heather, who is hearing impaired and must wear a hearing aid. The setting for the story is Heather's eighth birthday party. The narrative is enhanced by excellent colored photographs of Heather and others. This book could provide a basis for discussion of the effects of hearing loss on children's oral communication and thereby be instructive to all children in a classroom.

Baastad, B. F. (1965). *Kristy's courage*. New York: Harcourt, Brace, and World. (159 pages) (approximate **3rd grade readability** level)

Cheek and tongue injuries from being hit by a car leave Kristy with a scarred cheek and unclear speech. These problems are compounded by the fact that Kristy must start second grade in a new school. The big boys tease her and her classmates shun her. An understanding doctor helps the adults comprehend Kristy's problem and helps Kristy deal with it successfully.

Baldwin, D., & Lister, C. (1984). *You and your body. Your senses*. New York: The Bookwright Press. (32 pages) (approximate **6th grade readability** level)

Chapter 5 deals with the anatomy and function of the various parts of the ear. The text is written in simple language that can be understood by youngsters. Many colorful pictures illustrate points the authors wish to make. Suggestions are made on how to take care of one's ears.

Blatchford, C. (1976). *Yes, I wear a hearing aid*. New York: Lexington Family Series. (43 pages) (approximate **3rd grade readability** level)

Mumps caused the 6-year-old girl in this story to lose her hearing. The reader follows this girl from the time that she learns to cope with her first hearing aid as a 12-year-old through school, college, and parenthood.

Bloom, D. (1977). *The boy who couldn't hear*. London: The Bodley Head. (23 pages) (approximate **1st grade readability** level)

While fishing, Mark becomes frightened by some obviously angry boys who shout at him. His mother intervenes, explaining to the boys that Mark does not hear but lipreads instead. Amplification is briefly introduced in this picture book.

Bourke. L. (1981). *Handmade ABC. A manual alphabet*. Reading, MA: Addison-Wesley Publishing Company. (57 pages) (**picture book**)

This is a small book that is easy for little hands to grasp. The handshape for each letter is presented in clear black and white pictures.

Bove, L. (1980). *Sesame Street sign language fun*. New York: Random House. (62 pages) (**picture dictionary**)

Words and the signs for them (as presented by Linda Bove, a deaf actress on "Sesame Street") are arranged in concept families, such as family, morning, school, farm, playground, opposites, seasons, and feelings. Following each page of signs is a picture featuring the "Sesame Street" muppets and a sentence that the reader can practice signing.

Bove, L. (1985). *Sesame Street sign language ABC with Linda Bove*. New York: Random House. (29 pages) (**picture book dictionary**)

Linda Bove, a deaf actress on "Sesame Street," presents signs of words that begin with each letter of the alphabet. Other "Sesame Street" characters also appear in the book.

Broekel, R. (1984). *Your five senses*. Chicago: Children's Press. (48 pages) (approximate **4th grade readability** level)

How we hear is simply and clearly explained in large type in the hearing and sound chapter in this book. A glossary is included.

Brown, T., & Ortiz, F. (1984). *Someone special just like you*. New York: Holt, Rinehart and Winston. (64 pages) (picture book with captions at approximate **2nd grade readability** level)

This is a general book about being a special child. It is illustrated with numerous photographs. It emphasizes the point that children with disabling conditions are highly similar to other children in many respects. This book should be very helpful to the teacher who wants to educate all children about attitudes toward the disabled. An additional feature at the end of the book is the annotated bibliography that presents books, some written by disabled persons, that describe various disabling conditions.

Charlip, R., Beth, M., & Ancona, G. (1974). *Handtalk. An ABC of finger spelling and sign language.* New York: Four Winds Press. (40 pages) (**picture book**)

The handshape for each letter is presented along with the fingerspelling and sign for a word that begins with that letter.

Christopher, M. (1975). *Glue fingers.* Boston: Little, Brown and Co. (48 pages) (approximate **2nd grade readability** level)

Billy Joe is embarrassed by his stuttering, fears being laughed at, and feels that his stuttering interferes with his ability to make friends. Although he at first refuses to play football on an organized team because of his stuttering, Billy Joe finally rationalizes that he could join the team because he will not have to talk while playing. Happily, his prowess at football enables him to make friends with his teammates and to put his stuttering into perspective.

Corcoran, B. (1974). *A dance to still music.* New York: Atheneum. (180 pages) (approximate **4th grade readability** level)

Due to ear infections, Margaret becomes deaf while in eighth grade. Refusing to go to a school for the "handicapped," Margaret does not go to school at all. She lives in a silent, lonely world, refusing to try to talk for fear she will talk too loudly and harshly as her deaf grandmother had. When her mother plans to remarry, Margaret runs away and finds friendship with Josie and an injured Key deer. Events lead Margaret to talk again and agree to enter a university program designed to help deaf children learn to cope in a regular school.

Curtis, P. (1981). *Cindy: A hearing ear dog.* New York: E. P. Dutton. (55 pages) (approximate **6th grade readability** level)

Cindy, a small gray dog, is chosen from the animal shelter to be trained as a hearing ear dog. Such dogs help their hearing-impaired owners respond to various sounds, such as the telephone, door bell, alarm clock, and smoke detector. Lots of pictures explain the training process. At the end of the training period Cindy goes home with Jennifer, a deaf junior high student.

Elgin, K. (1967). *The human body: The ear.* New York: Franklin Watts. (49 pages) (approximate **5th grade readability** level)

Topics in this book include the variety of sounds that we can hear, the anatomy of the ear, how sound travels through the ear to the brain, and balance.

Emert, P. R. (1985). *Hearing ear dogs.* Mankato, MN: Crestwood House. (47 pages) (approximate **5th grade readability** level)

This book is very informative regarding hearing ear dogs. It begins with a story that shows the need for a hearing ear dog. A brief historical account is given of dogs who have helped hearing-disabled people in days gone by. A description is given of the breeds of dogs most frequently serving as helpers to deaf people. A most interesting section is the one on how these dogs are trained and then made available to their new masters. This book should be of interest not only to children but to parents as well. Edited by a professor of reading and language arts, it is well organized and interestingly written.

Fryer, J. (1961). *How we hear: The story of hearing.* Minneapolis, MN: Medical Books for Children: Lerner Publications. (30 pages) (approximate **7th grade readability** level)

The relationship of sound waves to pitch is explored. Then the author traces the path of sound from the time it enters the ear until it reaches the brain. Discussions of balance, motion sensitivity, and the purpose of the Eustachian tube are included. Possible causes of hearing problems and a brief description of hearing aids, including the first hearing aid used by Beethoven, conclude this book.

Gold, P. (1975). *Please don't say hello.* New York: Human Sciences Press. (47 pages) (approximate **3rd grade readability** level)

The neighborhood children are excited about the new family on their street. However, one of the three new children is a puzzle: Eddie is autistic. The neighborhood children learn that even though Eddie makes strange, eerie sounds and exhibits unusual behaviors, he is neither deaf nor retarded and will occasionally talk. Eddie is often afraid and confused and has difficulty concentrating. His feelings are hurt when he is teased. Additional information about autism is revealed through a visit to Eddie's school. Most importantly, the children learn that they can help Eddie by treating him naturally even though he does not respond as other children do.

Greenberg, J. E. (1985). *What is the sign for friend?* New York: Franklin Watts. (28 pages) (approximate **7th grade readability** level)

Lots of pictures are used to show Shane engaged in the ordinary everyday activities that children enjoy. Shane, who was born deaf, has difficulty learning to talk. His voice is sometimes high-pitched, he may omit sounds in words, and he is sometimes hard to understand. Shane has hearing friends as well as deaf friends. At school, he spends most of his day in classes with children who can hear. His interpreter signs the lessons for him and helps him keep up in his schoolwork. Signs for words, such as *friend, deaf,* and *pizza,* are given.

Greene, L., & Dicker, E. B. (1982). *Sign language.* New York: Franklin Watts. (66 pages) (approximate **8th grade readability** level)

The relationship between language and speech is briefly explained. Several sign language systems are introduced. The history of sign language includes a history of how hearing-impaired people have been viewed and treated through the years. A story (a Greek myth about the origin of the seasons) is told in words and sign. Sign language games can be found at the end of the book.

Hanlon, E. (1979). *The swing.* Scarsdale, NY: Bradbury Press. (209 pages) (approximate **5th grade readability** level)

Beth, who is deaf, is excited over the family's annual visit to the mountains. As Beth shares her many experiences—including coping with having to share her swing with Danny, hiking up the mountain for the first time by herself, and trying to save the bears—the reader learns that deafness has some limitations but certainly does not preclude talking or knowing that promises should be kept.

Haskins, J. S. (1978). *Who are the handicapped?* Garden City, NY: Doubleday and Company. (109 pages) (approximate **9th grade readability** level)

Several of the chapters in this book would be useful to teachers as they attempt to acquaint students with the concept of disability and the problems that are associated with being disabled. A special attempt is made by the author to address the prejudice often shown disabled people. Of particular interest are the sections on "Being Deaf" (pages 39–50) and "Cerebral Palsy" (pages 57–62).

Hirsch, K. (1981). *Becky*. Minneapolis, MN: Carol Rhoda Books. (35 pages) (approximate **2nd grade readability** level)

Becky, who is deaf, hears only very loud noises even with her hearing aid. She lives on a farm but stays with another family during the school week in order to go to a school where she can receive special help. The daughter of this family tells how she is surprised to find that Becky in many ways is just like other children. However, Becky is frustrated when she does not know how to communicate her thoughts. At her new school Becky learns how to use sign language and how to read lips, thus reducing that frustration. The two girls become good friends.

Hunter, E. F. (1963). *Child of the silent night*. Cambridge, MA: The Riverside press. (124 pages) (approximate **7th grade readability** level)

This is a compelling true story of a little girl, Laura, who became deaf and blind at the age of 2 following an illness. The daughter of farmers, this little girl was one of three children. Only limited time could be given to her as life on the farm in those days (nineteenth century) was very hard and demanding. Her real help came from a kindly neighbor man without a family who literally became her teacher. She was also helped by a student from Dartmouth who worked for Laura's father as a farmhand. It was through the help of this student, his professor, and others that Laura was enrolled in the Perkins Institution in Boston. Her progress was remarkable and she became known over the world. She lived at Perkins for 52 years and died at age 60.

Hyman, J. (1980). *Deafness*. New York: Franklin Watts. (64 pages) (approximate **10th grade readability** level)

Some infants are at high risk for hearing problems. Hyman discusses how it is often the parents who first notice that something seems to be wrong with their infant's hearing. How we hear; types of hearing loss; treatment, including surgery, medication, and hearing aids; ways for the hearing-impaired to communicate; mainstreaming; acceptance by peers; and difficulty with school tasks that require language, such as word problems in math, are among the topics explored.

Kamien, J. (1979). *What if you couldn't. . . . ? A book about special needs*. New York: Charles Scribner's Sons. (83 pages) (approximate **7th grade readability** level)

Kamien states that the purpose of this book is to help the reader understand more about various disabilities. One chapter addresses hearing loss. Lipreading, hearing aids, speech therapy, sign language, and total communication are presented as ways of coping with a hearing impairment. Other problems addressed in this book include visual impairments, learning disabilities, physical disabilities, emotional disturbance, and mental retardation.

Keller, H. (1954). *Helen Keller. The story of my life*. Garden City, NY: Doubleday and Company. (382 pages) (approximate **8th grade readability** level)

This is an autobiographical account of the life of Helen Keller. It outlines in detail the tremendous hurdles that Keller had to surmount as she worked with her dedicated and highly capable teacher, Anne Mansfield Sullivan. A supplementary report of her educational experiences is provided by her teacher. It is a splendid example of how a disabled person who is determined to learn can do so under the care of a knowledgeable and devoted teacher.

(NOTE: There are many accounts of Helen Keller's life written for many age levels and reading abilities.)

Kelley, S. (1976). *Trouble with explosives*. Scarsdale, NY: Bradbury Press. (117 pages) (approximate **3rd grade readability** level)

This story is told by a woman who is a stutterer. It exposes the many frustrations, fears, and anxieties caused by stuttering. It describes the reactions of her family and classmates. Written in a highly readable manner, it is laced with good humor and is hard to put down. This book should help students appreciate some of the difficult situations a stutterer must face.

Kettelkamp, L. (1967). *Song, speech, and ventriloquism*. New York: William Morrow and Company. (96 pages) (approximate **6th grade readability** level)

Voice production as a reflex action depends on the complex processes of respiration, phonation, and resonation. Each of these is explained in a straightforward manner. Production of many of the vowels and consonants is reviewed. Singing, breath control, voice ranges, and voice projection are explored, followed by a discussion on ventriloquism that uses the information learned about speech sound production. A glossary is included.

Krasilovsky, J. (1972). *The boy who spoke Chinese*. Garden City, NY: Doubleday and Co. (29 pages) (approximate **3rd grade readability** level)

Amanda explains to everyone that her younger brother, Nicholas, who doesn't speak clearly, is really speaking Chinese. Nicholas is frustrated because no one will listen and talk to him. Then he finds that his new baby brother is a very attentive listener. Some readers will be interested in knowing that this book was written and illustrated by a 15-year-old girl.

Lee, M. (1969). *The skating rink*. New York: Seabury Press. (126 pages) (approximate **6th grade readability** level)

Fifteen-year-old Tuck Faraday reacts to his stuttering problem with embarrassment and then withdraws from communicating. Befriended by Pete, who is building a skating rink in the rural town, Tuck learns to skate well enough to be an exhibition skater at the grand opening of the rink and to get a job giving skating lessons. With his newly found self-respect, Tuck decides that he does have a future after all and changes his mind about quitting school.

Levine, E. S. (1974). *Lisa and her soundless world*. New York: Human Sciences Press. (30 pages) (approximate **2nd grade readability** level)

This story helps the reader understand what it would be like not to be able to hear. Lisa did not learn to talk because she could not hear. When her parents discovered that she was deaf, they were able to get her help, which involved hearing aids and speech therapy, to learn to lipread, to talk, and to use sign language.

Litchfield, A. B. (1976). *A button in her ear*. Chicago: Albert Whitman and Co. (30 pages) (approximate **3rd grade readability** level)

This is a well-illustrated book for children that tells the story of a little girl, Angela, who has a hearing loss. Angela's hearing loss, identified by her parents, was further confirmed by her pediatrician, who sent her to an audiologist for further examination. This audiologist fitted her with a hearing aid that was of great help. This little book could be ever so helpful to other children who must wear hearing aids, and also to boys and girls in general, by giving them a better understanding and appreciation of children who must rely on hearing aids.

Litchfield, A. B. (1980). *Words in our hands*. Chicago: Albert Whitman & Co. (29 pages) (approximate **4th grade readability** level)

Nine-year-old Michael tells this story about his parents, who were born deaf, his two sisters, and their dog Polly. Michael and his sisters, who are not hearing impaired, learned sign language from their parents and speech from their grandparents, friends, and neighbors. Some of the topics worked into the story include fingerspelling, hearing ear dogs, teletypewriters, lipreading, and the National Theatre of the Deaf. Although embarrassment and shame are felt on occasion, the point is that Michael's family can take part in the same activities that other families do.

Litchfield, A. B. (1984). *Making room for Uncle Joe*. Niles, IL: Albert Whitman & Co. (26 pages) (approximate **2nd grade readability** level)

Uncle Joe has Down's syndrome and is coming to live with Danny, his younger sister Amy, his older sister Beth, and their parents. But how will he fit in? Will the children still be able to have their friends over to play? When they find that Uncle Joe listens to Amy read, teaches Dan to bowl, takes piano lessons from Beth, and helps around the house, he is accepted as a "neat guy."

Little, J. (1962). *Mine for keeps*. Boston: Little, Brown and Company. (186 pages) (approximate **4th grade readability** level)

This story is of a girl who returned home after having lived in a school for disabled children for over 5 years. Her fears at returning to her home are described. As a child with cerebral palsy, she knew that there would be many adjustments. Even though she had made two trips home each year for holidays, she sensed that coming home for good meant something different because others would have to adjust to her as well. The many situations described by the writer show the adjustments that can be made by a caring family and friends who understand.

MacIntyre, E. (1975). *The purple mouse*. New York: Thomas Nelson, Inc. (108 pages) (approximate **6th grade readability** level)

Because of four words that Hattie had been unable to hear, she manages to dye a white mouse a permanent purple. She has always believed that most people feel sorry for her because of her hearing impairment and so has just avoided people in general. However, in trying to help the little purple mouse, she learns to face her fears of difficult listening situations and to do as the purple mouse does—to never give up but to go forth.

McConnell, N. P. (1982). *Different and alike*. Colorado Springs, CO: Current. (28 pages) (approximate **6th grade readability** level)

The concepts of different and alike are used to emphasize the similarities between people who are and are not handicapped. Hearing and visual impairments, learning disabilities, speech disorders, and physical and mental handicaps are described. The book concludes with hints on how to help individuals with disabilities.

Martin, P. D. (1984). *Messengers to the brain. Our fantastic five senses*. Washington, DC: The National Geographic Society. (103 pages) (approximate **7th grade readability** level)

The chapter on hearing and balance provides a clear explanation of sound, how we hear, and how we maintain balance. The diagrams and pictures are excellent supplements to the text. A glossary is included.

Montgomery, E. R. (1978). *The mystery of the boy next door*. Champaign, IL: Garrard Publishing. (48 pages) (approximate **1st grade readability** level)

The neighborhood children think the new boy is very unfriendly when he ignores them and does not answer the doorbell. However, when they discover that both he and his mother are deaf, they understand how they reached the wrong conclusion, and a new friendship looms.

Peter, D. (1976). *Claire and Emma*. New York: John Day. (28 pages) (approximate **4th grade readability** level)

Claire and Emma, both born deaf, are 4 and 2 years old respectively. They live with their hearing mother and older brother. They both wear hearing aids and are learning to lipread. Pictures depict the usual childhood activities, such as swimming, climbing trees, and playing games that they enjoy. Some of the inconveniences of being hearing impaired, such as not being able to hear someone knock at the door, not hearing television, and not being able to lipread unless you are looking at a person, are highlighted.

Peterson, J. W. (1977). *I have a sister. My sister is deaf*. New York: Harper and Row. (29 pages) (approximate **4th grade readability** level)

The older sister tells in a gentle, loving manner what it is like to have a sister who is deaf. She tells how her sister is aware of what goes on around her even though she cannot hear. Even though the disadvantages of deafness are many, there are the occasional advantages, such as not being awakened and frightened by a thunderstorm.

Pollock, P. (1982). *Keeping it secret*. New York: G. P. Putnam's Sons. (110 pages) (approximate **2nd grade readability** level)

A sixth-grader, Mary Lou, better known as "Wisconsin," has just moved to New Jersey with her parents and brother. Wisconsin is fearful of meeting her new classmates because she wears hearing aids, so she tries to keep her aids a secret. This causes her classmates to misunderstand her actions. Field Day, a developing self-confidence, and Jason, who thinks she is cute, help her develop better social relationships.

Reuben, G. H. (1960). *What is sound*. Chicago: Benefic Press. (48 pages) (approximate **7th grade readability** level)

Sound is discussed in terms of the wide variety of sound sources, sound waves, the medium that carries sound waves, the speed of sound, breaking through the sound barrier, the frequencies and resulting pitches of sound, volume and the perceived loudness of sound, and sound reflections and echoes. The production of voice using expired air from the lungs and a short description of our uses of sound and how we hear complete the book.

Robinson, V. (1965). *David in silence*. Philadelphia: J. B. Lippincott Company. (126 pages) (approximate **6th grade readability** level)

The story is one of a boy, David, who was born deaf. It provides the reader with an excellent account of the many frustrating experiences David has in attempting to work out a place for himself among others as he develops. He is successful in changing the attitudes of classmates and others.

Rosen, L. D. (1981). *Just like everybody else*. New York: Harcourt Brace Jovanovich, Publishers. (155 pages) (approximate **3rd grade readability** level)

This is a story of a young girl, Jenny, who was deafened as a result of a bus accident. The writer describes with candor and clarity the many challenges Jenny has to meet in a silent world. The description of her struggle and eventual success in rehabilitation should deepen the student's understanding of deaf children. Because the author also lost her hearing, she is particularly sensitive to Jenny's problems.

Rosenberg, M. B. (1983). *My friend Leslie: The story of a handicapped child*. New York: Lothrop, Lee, and Shepard Books. (42 pages) (approximate **3rd grade readability** level)

Karin tells this story about her friend Leslie who is disabled. Leslie is visually impaired, has muscle stiffness, and is hearing impaired (she wears two hearing aids). Leslie can do most things for herself. It just takes her longer than it does the other children. At school Leslie is mainstreamed. Lots of pictures show what Leslie's school day is like in activities such as art, music, reading, and recess.

Rounds, G. (1980). *Blind outlaw*. New York: Holiday House. (94 pages) (approximate **7th grade readability** level)

Boy, who can only make a few sounds and cannot talk, has a special way of communicating with animals, including rabbits, coyotes, and a magpie. His challenge is to tame a wild blind horse. Boy seems to communicate with chirping and crooning noises, patience, and understanding. If he succeeds, the horse will be his.

Schneider, L. (1956). *You and your senses*. New York: Harcourt, Brace & World. (137 pages) (approximate **7th grade readability** level)

Experiments are suggested to reinforce the discussions of how sound is created, how sound travels, how the frequency and volume of sounds vary, how we hear, how the Eustachian tube functions, how we hear through bone, and how we maintain our sense of balance.

Schwartz, J. (no date). *A handful of colors*. Northfield, IL: cbh Publishing. (31 pages) (approximate **1st grade readability** level)

The signs for 57 high-frequency words are illustrated. Many of these signs are then repeatedly used in sentences that are also signed.

Showers, P. (1966). *How you talk*. New York: Thomas Y. Crowell. (35 pages) (approximate **1st grade readability** level)

In order to talk, people must use their lungs for a source of air, their vocal cords as a source of vibration, their teeth, tongue, lips, and so on. Talking is explored through humming with the nostrils opened and closed, changing the sound produced by changing the shape of the mouth, and trying to say words without using the tongue or the lips. The overall tone of the book is one of lightheartedness and fun.

Silverstein, A., & Silverstein, V. B. (1971). *The sense organs. Our link with the world*. Englewood Cliffs, NJ: Prentice-Hall. (73 pages) (approximate **7th grade readability** level)

One chapter of this book focuses on how we hear. Through the use of analogies, the anatomy and physiology of the ear are explained. How sounds may vary in pitch, loudness, and quality; how animals hear different pitches; and potential dangers to the hearing mechanism are touched upon.

Silverstein, A., & Silverstein, V. B. (1981). *The story of your ear*. New York: Coward, McCann, and Geoghegan. (64 pages) (approximate **7th grade readability** level)

The authors provide a relatively detailed explanation of the anatomy and physiology of the ear in an easy-to-understand manner. The frequencies and intensities of various sounds as they relate to hearing are explored. Noise as a source of potential damage to the ear and one's health and as an initiator of the flight-or-fight syndrome are discussed. This book is a good nonencyclopedic reference for a health or science report.

Slepian, J. (1980). *The Alfred summer*. New York: Macmillan Publishing. (119 pages) (approximate **3rd grade readability** level)

This is the story of a special friendship between "special" children. Cerebral palsy causes Lester to have problems with his speech and with walking. Alfred is mentally handicapped. Along with two other children, Lester and Alfred have their first experiences going places and doing things without a parent tagging along. At the end of one such outing, Lester must muster the strength to save his friend.

Smith, L. B. (1979). *A special kind of sister*. New York: Holt, Rinehart and Winston. (23 pages) (approximate **2nd grade readability** level)

Seven-year-old Sarah finds that it can be hard having a 5-year-old brother who is mentally handicapped. She shares with the reader her feelings and emotions regarding Andy, from jealousy over the attention that he requires to the empathy and love she feels.

Stanek, M. (1979). *Growl when you say R*. Chicago: Albert Whitman and Co. (29 pages) (approximate **2nd grade readability** level)

This is a story of an elementary school boy, Robbie, who had a problem articulating his "r" sounds. Because of this, he was teased by the other children. He got into fights and withdrew from play activities and his social development suffered. The teacher contacted the parents concerning Robbie's problem, and it was decided to send him to speech class. With reluctance Robbie went, and his efforts were rewarded by learning to say the "r" sound correctly. As a matter of fact, he was the child who was able to keep himself and some other children from becoming hopelessly lost at the zoo by being able to ask aloud over a microphone for his school bus driver to wait for them. The message was "Robert's School Bus Number 9 wait for us!"

Stecher, A., Wentworth, D. F., Couchman, J. K., & MacBean, J. C. (1973). *Your senses.* Toronto: Holt, Rinehart and Winston of Canada. (118 pages) (approximate **7th grade readability** level)

A variety of activities is outlined to help students better understand how we hear, how some people do not hear as well as others, how we identify sounds, how we localize sounds, how loud sounds affect our hearing, and so forth. Many of these activities are suitable for small groups.

Sullivan, M. B., & Bourke, L. (1980). *A show of hands—Say it in sign language.* Reading, MA: Addison-Wesley Publishing Company. (96 pages) (approximate **7th grade readability** level)

This book consists of a series of drawings that point out the importance and the use of hands by everyone in communicating ideas. It is a book not particularly to be read to student, but by them. It is suitable for adults as well. Signing and fingerspelling are explained through the narrative and through the drawings. This would be a good book to use in educating students as to how the hearing disabled are helped and would be particularly useful if a child in the classroom had a hearing impairment.

Talbott, M. (1982). *My treasure is my friend.* Northridge, CA: Joyce Media. (27 pages) (approximate **3rd grade readability** level)

David thinks the new boy next door is a snob. Then he learns that Chris ignores him because he is deaf and does not hear David's greetings. Chris and his mother help David learn about signing and lipreading. The two boys become good friends, even confronting a bully together. The next year at school the first words that Chris learns to speak are "My treasure is my friend David."

Wahl, J. (1978). *Jamie's tiger.* New York: Harcourt Brace Jovanovich, Inc. (43 pages) (approximate **3rd grade readability** level)

The author states that this book was written for both hearing-impaired and normal hearing youngsters to promote a better understanding between the two. A bout with German measles leaves Jamie hearing impaired and very lonely until, gradually, his friends become intrigued with signing and Jamie's ability to play the drums (he feels the rhythm).

Walker, L. A. (1985). *Amy: The story of a deaf child.* New York: Lodestar Books, E. P. Dutton. (59 pages) (approximate **3rd grade readability** level)

Eleven-year-old Amy and her parents are deaf. Her older brother is hearing. Pictures are used to show the normal activities, as well as those that are associated with a hearing impairment (e.g., how to use a teletypewriter-telephone, or TTY) that Amy engages in. At school Amy is in a regular classroom but also goes to see a speech-language pathologist and a teacher for the deaf for special help. There are two pages of resources at the end of the book.

Ward, B. R. (1981). *The ear and hearing.* New York: Franklin Watts. (40 pages) (approximate **9th grade readability** level)

With the help of colored diagrams the anatomy of the outer, middle, and inner ears is explained. Then the path of sound is followed from the time that it enters the outer ear until it is interpreted in the brain. How sound travels in waves, the range of sensitivity of the human ear, the ability to ignore unwanted sounds, the use of context to increase understanding, types of hearing loss, and how we maintain our balance are topics that are also included. A glossary is included.

Wolf, B. (1977). *Anna's silent world.* Philadelphia: J. B. Lippincott Company. (48 pages) (approximate **4th grade readability** level)

Illustrated with numerous pictures, this volume explains in a very graphic way all of the steps taken to help Anna, a 6-year-old who was born deaf, to lead a full life. Auditory training, lipreading, speech therapy, and adjustment to a hearing aid are just a few of the aspects of habilitation shown by the pictures. Students would learn a great deal about the problems and steps taken to help a child who is deaf.

Yolen, J. (1978). *The mermaid's three wisdoms.* Cleveland, OH: Collins World. (110 pages) (approximate **5th grade readability** level)

The mermaid Melusina is banned from the sea and given legs because she has allowed herself to be seen. Unable to talk because she has no tongue, Melusina is found by Jess, a hearing-impaired girl, and Captain A. Jess is able to communicate with Melusina by teaching her sign language. Through this experience Jess learns to better accept her hearing impairment and for the first time agrees to pull her hair back behind her ears (allowing her hearing aids to be seen) and proudly wear the earrings that Captain A promises to make from Melusina's crystal tears.

Zelonsky, J. (1980). *I can't always hear you.* Milwaukee, WI: Raintree Children's Books. (31 pages) (approximate **2nd grade readability** level)

This well-illustrated book is narrated by a little girl who wears a hearing aid. She relates the ways in which the hearing aid is helpful to her. Her misunderstanding of words at times is a source of amusement to classmates. An understanding teacher helps her by arranging a visit to the school principal, who also wears a hearing aid. As the little girl becomes better adjusted to others and the others to her, they all realize that there is something different about each of them—an allergy to chocolate, braces, no television at home, and so on. This is a book that should be helpful to all children in a classroom in which there is a child with a hearing loss.

Zim, H. S. (1956). *Our senses and how they work.* New York: William Morrow & Co. (64 pages) (approximate **6th grade readability** level)

A portion of this book explains the anatomy and physiology of the ear. The frequencies and loudness levels of various sounds are also discussed. Diagrams are used to supplement the text.

Some Additional Books to Consider

Almonte, P., & Desmond, T. (1992). *Learning disabilities*. New York: Macmillan Publishing. (48 pages) (for **grades 4–6**)

Various learning disabilities such as dyslexia, attention deficits, and processing problems are covered.

Amenta, C. (1992). *Russell is extra special: A book about autism for children*. Pasadena, CA: Magination Press. (for **grades 1–3**)

This illustrated book introduces an autistic boy and examines his problems, strange books, and play habits.

Baker, P. (1986). *My first book of sign*. Washington, DC: Gallaudet. (76 pages) (for **grades K–3**)

This is a beginning book on signing for use with those who wish to communicate with deaf people.

Bergman, T. (1989). *Finding a common language*. Milwaukee, WI: Gareth Stevens, Inc. (48 pages) (juvenile literature)

Follows the activity of a 6-year-old Swedish girl as she attends a nursery school for the deaf.

Dunn, K., & Boesel, A. (1993). *Trouble in school: A family story about learning disabilities*. Bethesda, MD: Woodbine. (for **grades 2–4**)

This book tells how a family dealt with their child's learning disability.

Fisher, G., & Cummings, R. (1980). *The survival guide for kids with LD (learning differences)*. Minneapolis, MN: Free Spirit. (for **grades 5–8**)

A supportive book aimed directly at kids with learning problems.

Isadore, R. (1985). *I hear*. New York: Greenwillow. (33 pages) (for **Preschool**)

Activities in a toddler's day depict familiar scenes.

Mathers, D. (1992). *Ears*. Mahwah, NJ: Troll Publishing. (for **grades 3–6**)

Explores the structures and functions of the outer, middle, and inner ear.

McCarthy-Tucker, S. (1993). *Coping with special-needs classmates*. New York: Rosen. (115 pages) (for **grades 5–8**)

First-person accounts describe physical, mental, and emotional problems faced by some young people.

McNamara, L. G., & Litchfield, A. B. (1973). *Your busy Brain*. Canada: Little Brown & Co. Ltd. (32 pages) (juvenile literature)

Describes the activity of the brain including sending and receiving messages, memory storage, learning, and creating.

Moragne, W. (1997). *Dyslexia*. Brookfield, CT: Millbrook Press, Inc. (96 pages) (juvenile literature)

Explains the nature of dyslexia, the various forms of treatment, and the many challenges faced by those living with this condition. Includes case studies and interviews.

Parker, S. (1989). *The ear and hearing*. Culver City, CA: Watts Publications. (40 pages) (for **grades 4–7**)

This account covers the anatomy of the ear and how it receives and transforms sounds.

Parker, S. (1992). *Singing a song: How you sing, speak, and make sounds*. Culver City, CA: Watts Publications. (32 pages) (for **grades 3–6**)

This book describes the various body parts required to create sounds.

Patterson, N. (1991). *The shiniest rock of all*. Greenville, SC: Farrar. (80 pages) (for **grades 3–5**)

Robert Reynolds cannot produce of all things—the letter *R*.

Rankin, L. (1991). *The handmade alphabet*. New York: Dial. (32 pages) (for **grades 4–9**)

Hands do the talking in this sign language alphabet book.

Roy, R. (1985). *Move over, wheelchairs coming through!* New York: Clarion Books. (83 pages) (juvenile literature)

Text and photographs present seven disabled youngsters between the ages of 9 and 13 who use wheelchairs in their fully active lives at home, at school, and on vacation.

Showers, P. (1990). *Ears are for hearing*. New York: Harper. (32 pages) (for **grades 2–4**)

The hearing process and parts of the ear are explained in this picture book.

Simon, C. (1990). *The boy of the bells*. New York: Doubleday and Company. (32 pages) (for **preschool–1**)

Aided by Santa Claus, Ben helps his sister regain her speech at Christmas time.

Taylor, B. (1989). *Living with deafness*. Culver City, CA: Watts Publications. (96 pages) (for **grades 5–8**)

Discusses causes of deafness and the ways people cope with this disability

Appendix *B*

Answers to Self-Test Questions

Chapter 1: Introduction to Speech, Language, and Hearing Problems in the Schools

1. an inflammation of the middle ear
2. a hearing loss
3. identify students who need an individual (or complete) evaluation
4. individualized educational program
5. least restrictive environment
6. classroom, curriculum (or vice versa)
7. monitoring, collaborative consultation, classroom-based, pullout, self-contained program, community-based, combination
8. stimulability
9. phonology, semantics, syntax, morphology, pragmatics
10. consultation or collaboration

1. False
2. False
3. False
4. True
5. False
6. False
7. False

8. False
9. False
10. True

Chapter 2: Articulation and Phonological Disorders

1. False
2. True
3. True
4. True
5. False
6. True
7. True
8. True
9. False
10. False
11. True
12. True
13. True
14. False

Chapter 3: Language Disabilities

1. False
2. Truc
3. True
4. False
5. False
6. Truc
7. False
8. False
9. True
10. True
11. False
12. True
13. False
14. False
15. False
16. True
17. False

18. False
19. True
20. True

Chapter 4: Stuttering

1. False
2. True
3. True
4. False
5. True
6. True
7. True
8. True
9. True
10. False
11. True
12. False
13. True
14. False
15. True
16. True
17. False
18. True
19. True
20. True

Chapter 5: Voice Disorders

1. True
2. True
3. True
4. False
5. True
6. True
7. True
8. False
9. False
10. True
11. False
12. True
13. False
14. True

15. False
16. True
17. False
18. True
19. False
20. False
21. True
22. False
23. True
24. True
25. False

Chapter 6: Hearing and Hearing Loss

1. B
2. C
3. B
4. C
5. A
6. D
7. D
8. A
9. A
10. B
11. C
12. D
13. D
14. C
15. C

Chapter 7: School Children with Hearing Impairments

1. True
2. True
3. False
4. True
5. False
6. False
7. True
8. False
9. False
10. False
11. True

12. False
13. False
14. False
15. True
16. True
17. True
18. True

Chapter 8: Low-Incidence Populations and Techniques of Special Concern

1. False
2. True
3. True
4. True
5. True
6. False
7. False
8. True
9. False
10. True
11. False
12. False
13. False
14. True
15. True
16. True
17. True
18. False
19. True
20. False
21. False
22. False
23. True
24. False
25. True

Index